PADMA

The book presents
the Jewel of Tibetan remedies
brought from the white peaks of the
Himalayas to the whole world
integrating ancient wisdom and
modern research using traditional
Tibetan herbs for today's diseases, and
harmonizing combinations of
vital substances.

PADMA

The Jewel of Tibetan Remedies

GABRIELE FEYERER

Translated by

CHRISTINE M. GRIMM

New Age Books

ISBN: 81-7822-220-5

First Indian Edition: Delhi, 2005

(First published 2003 by Lotus Press, USA)

Disclaimer:

The contents of this book have been carefully researched and reviewed. Despite this fact, we do not guarantee the validity of the information presented here. The author and publisher do not assume any type of liability for damages of any kind resulting from the application of the described remedies and procedures. Protected product names (trademarks) have not been specifically identified in the text. However, this does not mean that these are unknown product names. The implementation of all the information provided here is up to the free discretion of the reader. It is not intended as instructions for therapy. A medical diagnosis, as well as professional consultation, is always recommended; in no case does this book replace them.

Published by
NEW AGE BOOKS
A-44 Naraina Phase-I
New Delhi-110 028 (INDIA)
Email: nab@vsnl.in
Website: www.newagebooksindia.com

For Sale in South Asia Only

Printed in India
at Shri Jainendra Press
A-45 Naraina Phase-I, New Delhi-110 028

"AS AN INTEGRATED SYSTEM OF HEALTH CARE,
TIBETAN MEDICINE CAN OFFER ALLOPATHIC
MEDICINE A DIFFERENT PERSPECTIVE ON HEALTH.
HOWEVER, LIKE OTHER SCIENTIFIC SYSTEMS,
IT MUST BE UNDERSTOOD IN ITS OWN TERMS,
AS WELL AS IN THE CONTEXT
OF OBJECTIVE INVESTIGATION.
IN PRACTICE IT CAN ALSO OFFER WESTERN PEOPLE
ANOTHER APPROACH TO ACHIEVING
HAPPINESS THROUGH HEALTH AND BALANCE."

HIS HOLINESS THE DALAI LAMA

MAY 16, 1997

(Taken from the invitation
to the First International Congress for Tibetan Medicine
in Washington, 1998)

TABLE OF CONTENTS

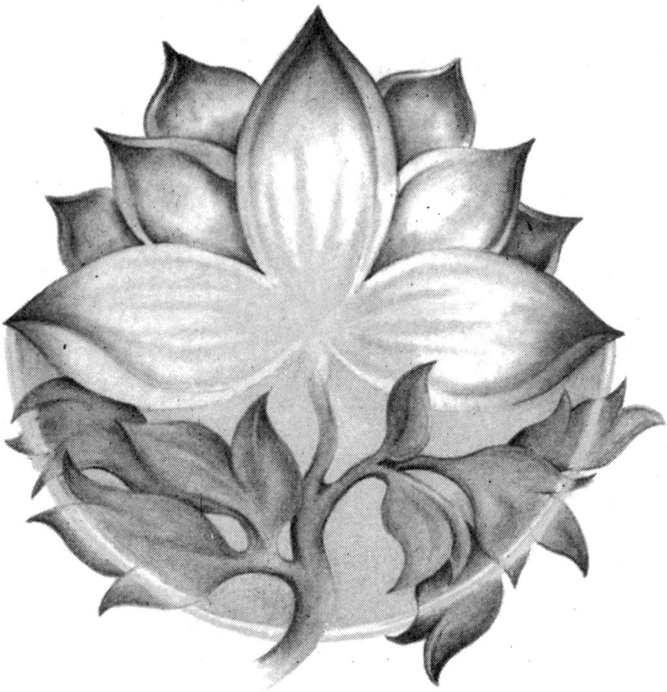

PREFACE

For the reader's information, I would like to begin with a few words of explanation.

I am not a physician, but an insightful devotee of medical correlations and the so-called naturopathy and folk medicine. I come from one of those traditional families whose grandmothers were accustomed to curing children's coughs with fennel honey and insect bites with a ribwort compress. I inherited both a love of nature and the healing power it holds. Moreover, my own experiences have shown the value and the possibilities of the Eastern systems of medicine.

This book is designed for readers who would like to have brief but rewarding overview of the principles of Tibetan medicine, as well as how its natural herbal remedies work. At the center of these considerations are two substance mixtures, which are being produced in the West for this first time under the name of *Padma*. However, other Tibetan formulas also follow the principle of variety in their ingredients. Plant remedies with many substances represent an aspect of the Tibetan medicine that distinguishes its practical applicability in a special way in the Western World. The formulas have been and continue to be subjected to internationally controlled medical studies for the purpose of distinctly documenting their effectiveness. Among other things, I want to describe the results of these test series for the interested readers in a generally understandable manner.

The information presented here does not claim to be complete, nor does this book aspire to be compared to scientific publications. Instead, it is intended to complement them. In this sense, if my work can make a contribution toward bringing the reader closer to the situation of Tibet, its human beings and its major tradition of medicine, this also gives me a sense of personal enrichment.

Gabriele Feyerer

INTRODUCTION: THE WISDOM OF THE MEDICINE-BUDDHA

Washington D.C., November 7, 1998: A group of Tibetan monks on the podium in a prayer position recited Buddhist texts. Slowly but surely, the auditorium filled. There were a total of more than 1600 physicians, scientists, press representatives and interested non-professionals attending the 3-day event.

His Holiness Tenzin Gyatso, the 14th Dalai Lama who lives in Indian Exile, held the formal opening speech for the **First International Congress for Tibetan Medicine**. This congress, he stated with a smile, was actually already the second international congress for Tibetan medicine: The first took place in the 8th Century and lasted 50 years.[1]

In a time frame that was naturally more limited, the Washington meeting offered participants from all over the world the new opportunity of exchanging their knowledge and practical experience. One main objective of the congress was the development of a dialog between the experts in the East and those in the West. The guiding motto for this was: "Revealing the Art of the Medicine-Buddha".

In his speech, the Dalai Lama said that we cannot permit the benefits of Tibetan medicine to be enjoyed only by Buddhists. In the same way, this body of knowledge must not remain closed to Western physicians.[2] In addition to a distinct rejection of obscure esoteric healing methods, the leader of Tibet also expressed his conviction that Tibetan medicine is effective independent of the Buddhist religion effective and a scientific study of the traditional medicinal formulas is desirable.

A BRIDGE BETWEEN CONTRASTING WORLDS

To a scientifically oriented physician, many aspects of Tibetan medicine may appear to be mysterious and mystical. Yet, there has long been a Tibetan formula in Europe, which was produced for the first time on a trial basis in 1965 in Switzerland and has since awakened great interest among scientists and practitioners from many countries. This is a natural herbal preparation with the name of *Padma 28,* which is now called Padma Basic in the USA and other nations. Numerous research results have since confirmed the health advantages of this Tibetan medicine formula. At the congress in Washington, interesting new studies and user reports were presented.

So what is Tibetan medicine actually about? How does it work, and when can you use such standardized multiple-substance mixtures for your health? Where can you find more information? These and similar questions are frequently asked. Please continue reading for their answers!

TIBETAN MEDICINE—
THE KNOWLEDGE OF HEALING

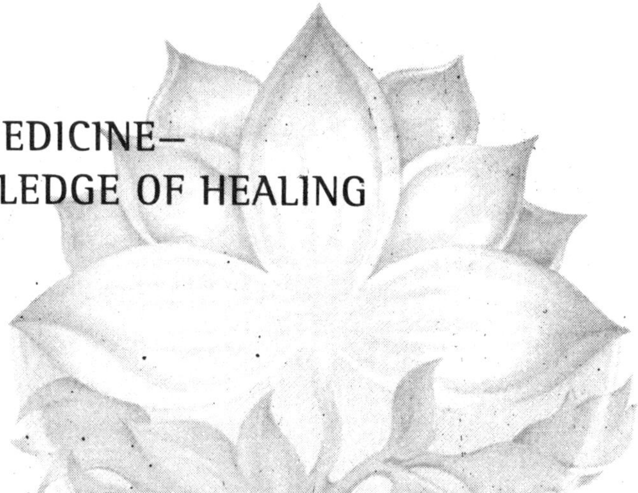

The autonomous region of Tibet, which today is under the rule of China, is located on the high Tibetan plateau, often called the "Roof of the World." The traditional medicine of the Tibetans is among the oldest of the continually practiced healing traditions in the world. This system is more than 2000 years old and is fascinating because of its logic and holistic approach.

Despite its turbulent fate, Tibetan medicine has been successfully practiced through many centuries in the Himalayan areas, parts of China, Mongolia, and other Buddhist-influenced regions of Asia.

Since it is inseparably connected with the Buddhist worldview, Tibetan medicine has a completely different characteristics and another orientation than our Western system. It is more than just a collection of facts—as medicine for the body, mind and soul, it shows us the "path to the right way of living."

AN EVENTFUL HISTORY

Beginning with the shamanic Bon tradition, a medical tradition has existed in Tibet since time immemorial. With the introduction of Buddhism and the Tibetan script in the 7th Century A.D. by King Songtsen Gampo, this medical knowledge was associated with Chinese, Indian and Persian-Hellenic sources. In the year 800, a meeting of Asian medical experts took place for the first time under Yutog Yonten Gonpo the Elder, the personal physician to the Tibetan king. According to the old traditions, they discussed, compared, and developed an independent Tibetan medical system from a combination of the best texts.

The initial translation of the fundamental reference work of Tibetan medicine, later called **"The Four Tantras"** (*Gyueshi = rgyud-bzhi)* by the famous scholar and translator Vairochana.

Yutog Yonten Gonpo the Younger was considered to be the greatest Tibetan physician of all times and the 14th incarnation of the Medicine-Buddha. In the 12th Century, he put "The Four Tantras" into their current definitive form. In 156 chapters and 5900 verses, this medical work describes 1600 illnesses and 2293 remedy ingredients. In addition to many other writings, "The Four Tantras" were supplemented by the commentary **"Blue Beryl"** in the 17th Century. The 5th Dalai Lama, who was considered to be the unifier of Tibet and great supporter of the medicine, additionally commissioned 79 **thangkas** (scroll paintings), which were meant to visually depict the text of the commentary as a type of medical atlas. Even today, studying these pictures is still an important component in the training of every Tibetan physician.

THE DEVELOPMENT OF THE MEDICAL SCHOOLS

In Lhasa, the capital of Tibet, the Potala Palace was built as the new winter headquarters of the Dalai Lama at the same time as the medical school **Chagpori** ("Iron Mountain") as the center of monastic scholarship. In the 18th and 19th centuries, other medical schools were founded according to the model in Lhasa, including those in Peking and Mongolia. The physicians trained there called themselves *menpa* or *amchi* (Mongolian). In Siberian Buryatia (Transbaikalia) as well, Tibetan medicine became widespread through Buddhism. According to the tradition, the Tibetan physician Sultim Badma and his descendents later brought their knowledge as far as Russia and Europe.

In 1916, the 13th Dalai Lama the *Men Tsi Khang* (*Men* = medicine, *Ts*= astrology, *Khang* = house) was founded in Lhasa. Laymen were admitted to the medical studies for the first time here. However, Tibet experienced radical changes in the second half of the 20th century.

THE ANNEXATION OF TIBET

Tibet has always had to defend itself against the superior force of China. Although the country has an autonomous status, this is not backed by the safeguards of international law. Already in 1936, Tibetan medicine was prohibited in Mongolia by the Soviets and all traces of it were almost completely eradicated. In 1949, Tibet was annexed by the newly created People's Republic of China. Under the pretext of "social and cultural assistance," this was followed by an era of the systematic exploitation and suppression of the Tibetan people. After futile efforts of achieving peace, the 14th Dalai Lama, the religious and political leader of Tibet, saw himself forced to flee to India with about 100,000 followers. He established an exile government there in the small Indian village of Dharamsala.

In Lhasa, the hostilities soon reached their climax. The *Men Tsi Khang* was closed and the medical school *Chagpori* was razed to the ground. Almost all of the Tibetan monk-physicians were arrested, tortured and many of them murdered. Countless valuable medical writings became victim to the fury of the Chinese invaders and the so-called "cultural revolution." Since this time, 1.2 million Tibetans have died through hunger, persecution, and other life struggles.

For his sincere efforts at achieving peace and understanding, H.H the Dalai Lama was honored with the Nobel Peace Prize in 1989

Although China suspended its martial law over Tibet in 1990, life became more and more difficult for the Tibetans. Tibetan areas were systematically settled by the Chinese. Today, the Tibetans are a minority within their own country. Despite propaganda to the contrary, free expression of opinions and practice of religion are hardly tolerated in the practice. The curriculum at the reopened *Men Tsi Khang* is closely monitored on the part of the Chinese. In many Western nations, there are now organizations that help Tibet by supporting and preserving the identity of the uprooted Tibetan people (see page 149). New opportunities have also arisen from the increased spread of Buddhism to Western countries during recent years.

TIBETAN MEDICINE IN EXILE

In order to preserve the traditional healing knowledge, H.H. the Dalai Lama established a medical school in 1961 in Dharamsala. The mission of the Tibetan Medical & Astrology Institute (now called *Men Tsee Khang*) is to preserve and spread the tradition of Tibetan medicine and train physicians, as well as ensure generally affordable health care. The *Men Tsee Khang* has a hospital with branches throughout all of India, a pharmacy and other departments, such as those for the production of medicinal remedies and research. Patients from around the world can directly contact the *Men Tsee Khang* with their medical diagnosis in order to obtain the respective Tibetan medicines from it (see appendix for details).

WESTERN MEDICINE AS A BLESSING AND A BURDEN

In the Traditional Hospital of the Autonomous Region of Tibet, many of the physicians now are also skilled at Western medicine, which is an advantage for their patients. Yet, this enrichment can also be a disadvantage. Buddhism as the foundation of the teachings of Tibetan medicine is being sometimes pushed into the background.

Without consideration of its Buddhist roots and the Tibetan culture, I believe that a deeper understanding of Tibetan medicine is hardly possible. However, as H.H. the Dalai Lama has repeatedly emphasized, it is effective independent of the religion. The objective examination of the teachings of Tibetan medicine should therefore not lead to Westernization but to its appreciation as an independent and equal system. Scientific studies of Tibetan remedies, as they are currently taking place throughout the world, do not contradict this objective in any way. It is also obvious that Tibetan physicians must carefully monitor this modernization process.

Today, centers for Tibetan medicine exist not only in Asia, but also in some of the European countries. In many of them, a Tibetan physician is always present. In addition, visits by Tibetan "wandering physicians" to the West are organized on a regular basis.

However, the tendency of Tibetan physicians to go to the West is momentous for their own people. After training that lasts about two decades, many of them decide to remain in Western countries because the living conditions are better. As a consequence, their home region is robbed of a great intellectual potential. Tibetan physicians can no longer be found in many of the northern Indian monasteries.

In 2001, Tibetan medicine lost a truly great master in Dr. Tenzin Choedrak, the late personal physician of H.H. the 14th Dalai Lama.

HEALTH AND ILLNESS FROM THE TIBETAN PERSPECTIVE

According to the legend, the historic Buddha Shakyamuni brought the art of healing to human beings. In the concept of the physician as the Medicine-Buddha, this belief reveals the close intertwining of healing knowledge and religious teachings. According to the Buddhist philosophy, the universe is in a perpetual state of flow. The only constant element is inconsistency. Furthermore, the concept of reincarnation is at the center of the Tibetan view of life. Human life is characterized by suffering, whereby our own ego blindness leads to unrestrained desires and negative thinking.

ILLNESS BEGINS AND ENDS IN CONSCIOUSNESS

In Tibetan medicine, the human mind is seen as the foundation of all phenomena. It determines health and illness. The prescribed medicine is only one part of the spiritual path *(dharma)*, through which our entire being can be purified and harmonized. An essential aspect of Tibetan medicine is the comprehensive understanding of psychosomatic correlations. This is also an emanation of the philosophy of Buddhist beliefs, in which benevolent understanding and compassion with all beings are highly valued.

Wrong thinking is considered to be the long-term cause of illnesses, whereby the **"Three Poisons of the Mind"** (attachment and desire, aversion, and ignorance) play a major role. Other causes are improper diet and lifestyle, as well as negative environmental influences. However, from the Buddhist perspective, human suffering is created by unethical deeds in past lives ("karmic burdens") and even through the work of evil demons. The treatment of such illnesses is considered to range from difficult to impossible.

HEALTH MEANS EQUILIBRIUM

Everywhere in the world, ancient medical systems agree in their statements about the nature of health and illness. They have in common the conviction that body, soul, and mind form an inseparable unity. Health means maintaining a dynamic equilibrium of the universal elemental forces. Illness and suffering are dissonances in this cosmic harmony.

According to the teachings of Tibetan medicine, the body—and the universe in general—consists of the five "elements" of Earth, Water, Fire, Wind (air), and Space, which penetrates everything else. Each of these **elements** exercises a very specific influence on the life functions of the body. Illnesses manifest themselves through an imbalance of the three body energies or body fluids of **"Wind," "Bile," and "Phlegm."** However, these terms should not be understood in the Western sense; instead, they describe various processes in the human organism. The separation into **cold and hot illnesses** makes it possible to gain further conclusions about the cause and reason for a disorder. In this teaching, imbalances of Wind and Phlegm are considered cold disorders, but Bile disorders and "impure blood" are seen as hot diseases. This description, which is naturally very simplified, makes it adequately clear that Tibetan medicine is a holistic system that does not search only for the symptoms of the ailment but also attempts to treat its actual causes.

The ancient medical writings use the following example to illustrate this approach: When the causes of an illness are not eliminated, it is as if just the leaves and twigs are trimmed from a poisonous tree without also tearing up the roots. It is certain that it will continue to grow.

DIAGNOSIS AND THERAPY

Tibetan physicians practice a special technique of feeling the pulse as the fundamental means of diagnosis. The masters of this specialty can distinguish between 48 different pulse qualities.

When a Tibetan physician "reads" the wrist pulse of his patient, he uses it to determine (among other things) the blood flow that is connected with the Wind energy. Since the energy of Wind is the principle of the body that moves everything, the condition of all the organs and the type of existing fluid disorder can be recognized. The emotional-mental condition of the sick person is reflected in his or her body "fluids." It is quite astonishing to see how a practitioner of Western medicine reaches the same conclusions after complicated tests that his Tibetan colleague achieves after feeling the pulse for 2-3 minutes. There is hardly an approach that is less expensive, yet so efficient.

INSIGHT AND DHARMA

In most cases, the Tibetan physician only requires the pulse diagnosis with a brief questioning of the patient to come up with a fundamental diagnosis. When there is a lack of clarity and a complicated fluid disorder, this is also followed with an analysis of the urine, eyes, skin, and tongue. The insights of the sick person as to what part he or she has played in the affliction–where he or she has left the path of *dharma* from the Buddhist perspective–is important for a successful treatment. And this is actually where most health problems can be either directly or indirectly traced back to improper nutrition, combined with stress and afflictive emotions. Each therapy should therefore begin at these points. However, today Tibetan medicine usually begins with the formula of healing herbal preparations since a change in life circumstances is very difficult to initiate in most patients.

Tibetan medicine, in as far as it is correctly selected and the disorder is properly recognized, eliminates not only the symptoms of an illness but also simultaneously heals its causes. This is a total contrast to Western pharmacy, the remedies of which are always primarily aimed at the elimination of symptoms. The medicinal remedies or inner therapy is supplemented from case to case by external measures such as moxibustion (burning of mugwort herb above specific parts of the body), cupping, bloodletting, or acupuncture with a thick gold needle. Some of these methods are not particularly "gentle," but they are apparently very effective for severe illnesses. In addition, Buddhist patients are told to support the treatment through meditation, prayers, and visualizations.

TIBETAN MEDICINE WORKS INDEPENDENTLY

The treatment with Tibetan remedies always develops its special effects—no matter whether the physician and/or patient is Buddhist or not. A Tibetan monk-physician will always accompany his treatment with prayers because this corresponds with the religious sensibility of this culture. When a Western medical practitioner encounters his patients with benevolence and friendly gestures, he does something very similar.

Of course, Tibetan medicine cannot and should not replace Western medicine. This should be emphasized here because each has a very different set of strengths and qualities. But both systems can very meaningfully complement each other. Tibetan medicine has proven to be especially successful in the treatment of chronic ailments. So in the daily practice, it may often be at least as effective as our Western system—and, above all, it would cost less. However, patients who are hoping for a quick solution to health problems that have usually developed over the course of many years may be disappointed. Tibetan herbal medicines, for example, must be taken over a longer period of time before the initial success is visible because they generally provide gentle healing impulses. The Buddhist philosophy of life is also reflected here: Without patience, a bit of humility and the will to change, the desired equilibrium will not occur.

TIBETAN REMEDIES–EXPERIENCE OF THOUSANDS OF YEARS

Tibetan medicine has a great variety of ingredients for the production of inner remedies: plants, trees, resins, minerals and earths, precious metals, and many more. According to the universal laws, literally anything that exists can become a remedy. However, about 95% of the traditional medicine formulas are based on plant material. The gentlest type of treatments in Tibetan medicine are those with decoctions of pulverized plants; these are followed by powders, syrups, and finally compressed herbal pills.

HERBAL AND JEWEL PILLS

The plants required for Tibetan medicinal remedies are primarily gathered in the upper reaches of the Himalayas and evaluated for their specific active-substance profile according to the location. For example, plants that grow in the sun and at lower levels commonly have warming or heating qualities. Accordingly, they are applied against cold disorders. On the other hand, shade plants and those from high altitudes commonly have a cooling effect, which heal heat disorders. The time they were gathered, how they were processed, and even astrological influences play a role, as well as which parts of the plant are used.

In Lhasa and Dharamsala, the production of herbal medicines occurs strictly according to the ancient tradition. Improved effects and tolerance are guaranteed in this case. The main problem continues to be the limited sources of raw substances and the difficult financial situation of both centers.

HEALING POWER WITHOUT SIDE EFFECTS

Contrary to the Western perspective, Tibetan medicine assumes that even a simple medicine can also be harmful. A plant that has a useful effect on a specific organ of the body will almost always have a negative effect on others at the same time. For this reason, only about 80% the components in Tibetan medicine are aimed at healing the pathological disorder while the rest of the substances in the mixture are intended to ward off any undesired side effects.

Tibetan herbal pills contain up to 35 various ingredients in very small dosages each. Unfortunately, many plants of the Himalayan region are currently threatened by extinction. Although the use of similar species from other high-mountain areas is being considered, whether they will ensure the same type of success is questionable. Even naming the approximately 1000 various plants, of which 300 to 400 are continuously in use, is puzzling because most of them only have Tibetan names.

TASTE AS AN INDICATOR

The essential criterion of a Tibetan medication is its taste. From the interaction of the five elements, **six** recognizable **taste directions** are distinguished in foods and remedies. These six taste directions must be eaten on a regular basis and in a balanced relationship to each other in order for us to remain healthy.

There are also additional "qualities," "potencies," and "post-digestive tastes" that are important for the composition of the medicinal remedies. The taste of an herbal pill will make it possible to quite exactly predict the direction of its effect. A compound medicine that fulfills all of the taste requirements would practically be a universal remedy in the hands of the knowledgeable physician, capable of eliminating any type of fluid disorder.

PRECIOUS PILLS

A specialty of Tibetan medicine is the jewel pills or precious pills. On the one hand, they are taken to maintain good health; on the other hand, these medicines can have an immune-strengthening and restorative effect, healing all types of disorders. In contrast to the usual herbal pills, the medicinal plants for the jewel pills are not dried but boiled to a mush. Then sulfur, powdered gemstones, minerals, and metals are added to it. This hardly meets the standards of medicinal safety required in the West, which is why general distribution cannot be permitted. After the respective diagnosis, jewel pills must be prescribed by a physician trained in Tibetan medicine and should come from reliable sources! There are currently **seven types of jewel pills** being produced in Dharamsala, containing between 25 and 165 individual components. They bear a special seal of quality.[3]

According to the ancient Tibetan sources, jewel pills are called the medicine for the newly occurring illnesses of coming generations. Dr. Tenzin Choedrak, the former personal physician to the Dalai Lama tested the effects of the jewel pills with great success on the victims of the Chernobyl catastrophe. Aids patients could also benefit from the jewel pills.[4]

However, the creation of this very valuable medicine is currently only possible to a limited degree because of the lacking raw substances and financial means. The complicated production process, which is still secret in part, does not permit any type of true mass production.

THE VOICE OF SCIENCE

"Our healing arts must stand up to a critical analysis ..." is how H.H. the Dalai Lama underlined his request on the occasion of the Washington congress for a suitable study program to make the Tibetan "knowledge of healing" understandable and applicable for us in the West.[5] However, the path there is still quite rocky and paved with major obstacles.

NARROWNESS VERSUS DIVERSITY

Tibetan medicinal remedies are carefully composed multi-substance mixtures that do not fit within the scope of the usual scientific descriptions. This factor is what precisely makes their recognition so difficult. Our modern pharmacology namely strives to dissect each individual plant into its effective components, then isolate them and chemically reproduce them. Pharmaceutical companies throughout the world are constantly searching for mono-substances, meaning individual substances that they can patent and from which they can earn their profits. But such an approach is not possible with Tibetan medications.

Michael McIntyre, a specialist for phytotherapy and the director of the *Midsummer Cottage Clinic* in England, speaks of "allopathic raisin-picking" to point out how even interested physicians usually just use individual plants in their practice and prescribe them like any other drugs. However, the basis of plant medicine, McIntyre emphasizes, is the idea of variety: the **poly-pharmacy.**[6] What is the purpose of reducing the entire organism of the plant to the chemical reaction of a few of its molecules?

THE ERROR OF LINEAR THOUGHT PATTERNS

The Viennese biophysicist Dr. Herbert Schwabl has done detailed research on *Padma Basic's* mechanism of action (see the Chapter "Padma Basic—Motor of the Immune System"). Along with many other people, he is convinced that the future belongs to the non-linear sciences.[7]

Non-linear thought means that not every effect can be immediately associated with a tangible cause. Non-linear thinking demands more farsightedness and a holistic view of things. This means leaving the well-beaten scientific paths to gain deeper insights into the functioning of complex systems, which is also what the human body is. This is a path that folk medicine has always taken.

For medical research and practice, this approach means: We must be willing to recognize the apparent overall effect of the Tibetan multi-substance mixtures, as it has clearly come to light in test series—without wanting to duplicate it down to the last detail. As a result, there is little sense in carrying out a complicated analysis of the individual biochemical processes. Increasing more illnesses are now being triggered by a multitude of factors (diet, lifestyle, environment, etc.). This makes the idea of encountering them with a multitude of substances even more obvious. In terms of the healing potential of Tibetan mixtures of effective substances, the sum of 2 plus 2 may very well be more than four.

TIBETAN MEDICINE AS AN INFORMATION CARRIER

As we now know, an individual component never dominates in a Tibetan formula; instead, it is only the combination of selected components that creates their frequently astounding overall effect. Each of these complex structures of active substances supplies the body with a multitude of impulses in the direction of health, helping it to return to its natural equilibrium. Tibetan remedies serve as messages that the organism understands and independently translate into action. In this process, the smell and taste of a medicine are just as important as the time period in which it is taken. Each factor fits with the other like the pieces of a puzzle. It would be impossible, as well as senseless, to want to attribute the healing power of such mixtures to a single active principle.

BEYOND BOOK LEARNING

To clarify the question as to why Tibetan medicine functions in this way and not in another, our rational science is still largely lacking in the necessary qualifications. As H.H. the Dalai Lama explained in an interview with the film director Franz Reichle, there is a group of Tibetan medications whose characteristics are dependent upon certain natural phenomena, among other things. They are only completely effective when, for example, they are subjected to the light of the full moon. Even precise astrological calculations in the production or ingestion can be decisive for the healing power of a specific medicine.[8]

The Tibetans call this phenomenon of cosmic dependencies *tendrel* and consider it to be completely obvious. A comparable effect can perhaps be seen in Western homeopathy in the medicines "Sol" and "Luna."* Their effectiveness is also based on metaphysical sources. We now know that the benefits and side effects of pharmaceutical drugs can be changed depending upon the time of ingestion. This

* Milk sugar is subjected to the sun or moon light and becomes a completely effective medication. "Sol" is highly effective for instance against effects of sun-burn. This remedy contains "nothing" besides light.

evolving field is called chronobiology. It is very useful in the administration of chemotherapeutic drugs.

Our "book learning" is still at a loss when it comes to this approach—unfortunately.

However, as the Dalai Lama emphasized at the Washington congress, the origins of Tibetan medicine are scientific, even if they are in part out of the reach of the research common to the West.

For the same reason, Dr. Namgyal Qusar of the *Men Tsee Khang* Institute in Dharamsala advocates a "participating observation" of the work of Tibetan physicians, without solely evaluating their success according to our criteria. Yet, the openness of the Tibetans for cooperation is obvious, and the West should take advantage of this offer —according to Robert A. Thurman from the *University of Columbia.*

PADMA BASIC– MESSENGER OF A GENTLER MEDICINE

KARL LUTZ DISCOVERS TIBETAN MEDICINE

In Zurich, during 1954: The Swiss pharmaceutical Vice President of Research Karl Lutz listened spellbound to the lecture by a Benedictine father about Tibetan medicine.

He was fascinated by what he heard and became interested in this ancient medical teaching.

Through the speaker, Father Cyrill von Korvin-Krasinski, Karl Lutz became acquainted with the Polish surgeon Peter Badmajew. The latter's deceased father, Vladimir Badmajew, had adopted the Tibetan medicine from his famous Buryat (eastern Mongolian) ancestors and continuously applied it successfully in his Warsaw physician's practice in addition to the Western approach. The late Vladimir Badmajew was the last trained Tibetan doctor of his family. His estate also included a description of Tibetan medicine formulas. The Polish state and the pharmaceutical companies showed absolutely no interest in them, but Karl Lutz had a premonition of the treasure that was handed over to him. He had some of the medicines produced on a trial basis. The Study Group for Tibetan Medicine in Zurich (with Karl Lutz as the main driving force) worked out a precise, at that time unique list of indications for all 14 traditional formulas. The entire series was made available to interested physicians. It was very fortunate that Karl Lutz could rescue the unique Tibetan heritage from falling into oblivion in post-Stalinist Poland.

A FORMULA BECOMES A HOUSEHOLD NAME

For his medicines, Karl Lutz selected the name *Padma*. (In Sanskrit, this word stands for the lotus blossom, the symbol of purity and beauty.) The indications for Formula No. 28 attracted his attention. Padma 28 (or Padma Basic, as it is called in the USA) proved to be surprisingly effective in the treatment of arterial occlusion diseases, such as the well-known smokers' leg. Increasing more patients reported on an astonishing improvement of their complaints, which were more permanent than with vasodilating medications. Studies were conducted, which then confirmed the observed effects of Padma Basic.[9] The production technique was improved to make the Tibetan tablets according to strict Swiss quality. By 1978, Padma Basic was approved as an over-the-counter medication in Switzerland.

However, the path to its official acceptance as a medication by Swiss health insurance companies in March of 1998 was a long one paved with bureaucratic hurdles. The reservations and resistance against it were major on the part of orthodox medicine. Yet, Karl Lutz fought untiringly for his convictions. He is credited with having been the first to comprehend the significance of Tibetan medicine and setting the decisive course for the recognition of Tibetan remedies in Europe.

His life's work is being continued by the Swiss pharmaceutical company **Padma, Inc.**, whose founder and director he was until his death in 1995. *Padma* has always been a research-oriented company dedicated to the production of high-quality Tibetan formulas. It sponsors the largest research program for Tibetan formulas in the world.

Using the original composition and strict quality control, the company produces the two formulas Padma Basic and Padma Lax in Switzerland, as well as four Tibetan tea mixtures (for more information on this, see the chapter "Tibetan Teas—A Simple Way to Achieve Well-Being"). Fourteen additional *Padma* formulas have recently been admitted in the Swiss canton of Appenzell Ausserrhoden.

WHY PADMA BASIC WORKS

Even during the time when the formulas of the physician family of Sultim Badma traveled through the Mongolia and Russia to Europe, many of the herbs from the high Himalayas were probably replaced with similar specimens from the native plant world. As a result, the Tibetans themselves are somewhat suspicious of the formula Padma Basic. However, the current formula was checked for its perfect composition by Dr. Donden, the founder of the *Men Tsee Khang* in Dharamsala and evaluated to be correct.

Padma Basic is a typical representative of the gentle Tibetan plant medicine. The compressed herbal tablets consist of 21 natural components, 19 of them plants and parts of plants, in connection with natural camphor and calcium sulfate. Overall, this results in a content of more than 10,000 different substances that interact **synergistically**, meaning that they combine and mutually strengthen each other. The plant parts in Padma Basic are finely milled to powder, but are otherwise left in their raw state.

The components of Padma Basic can be divided into three different actions according to the principles of Tibetan medicine:

1. Components that determine the main effect
2. Components that support this effect
3. Components that counteract the undesired effects of the other components.

Contents of Padma Basic

Scientific Name	Common Name	Milligram (mg) per Tablet	Essential Oils	Tannins	Bitter substances	Saponins (nitrogen-free glycosides)	Polysaccharides (Mucogenics)	Flavonoids (col. substances of flowers and blossoms)
Ce Cetraria islandica	Iceland Moss	40					•	
Saussurea costus	Costus root	40	•					
Azadirachta indica	Neem fruit	35			•			
Elettaria cardamomum	Cardamom fruit	30	•					
Pterocarpus santalinus	Red saunders	30	•					
Terminalia chebula	Chebulic Myrobalan	30		•				
Pimenta dioica	Allspice fruit	25	•					
Aegle marmelos	Beal tree fruit	20					•	
Calcium sulfate	Gypsum	20						
Aquilegia vulgaris	Columbine herb	15						•
Plantago lanceolate	English plantain herb	15					•	•
Glycyrrhiza glabra	Licorice root	15				•		
Polygonum aviculare	Knotweed herb	15						•
Potentilla aurea	Golden Cinquefoil herb	15		•				•
Syzygium aromaticum	Clove flower bud	12	•					
Hedychium spicatum	Spiked gingerlily rhizome	10	•			•		
Sida cordifolia	Heart-leaf sida herb	10					•	•
Valeriana officinalis	Valerian root	10	•					
Lactuca sativa	Wild lettuce leaf	6						•
Calendula officinalis	Calendula flower	5						•
Cinnamomum camphora	Camphor	4						

Source: EcoNugenics, Inc. (see page 149)

These rules are observed in the composition of every kind of Tibetan herbal medicine.

A look at the components of Padma Basic (see table) reveals that this formula unexpectedly consists not only of plants coming from Tibet and Southeast Asia. Instead, we come across such "common" well-known plants like ribwort, knotgrass, or cinquefoil. Yes, even leaves of lettuce (Lactuca sativa) are contained in it. Only a portion of the plant contained in Padma Basic are actually exclusively found in Asian countries; the rest can also be found in other areas. Icelandic moss is only native to Northern Europe, for example. The ingredients for Padma Basic are now purchased by the manufacturing company from the specialized market for medicinal herbs. Where possible, the plant materials come from Swiss controlled organic cultivation.

THE BITTER PILL

As explained above, the smell and taste of a medicine plays a decisive role in Tibetan medicine. In relation to Padma Basic, just these properties alone allow conclusions about the spectrum of effects.

Padma Basic tastes bitter, somewhat pungent and penetrating. According to the teachings of Tibetan medicine, it therefore has cooling qualities. The formula stimulates the energy of Wind, as well as Phlegm to a lesser degree. It has a soothing effect on Bile. This means that its beneficial effects should be found in the areas of "heat disorders" such as inflammations, cardiovascular disease, arteriosclerosis, chronic infections, and immunodeficiencies. In the meantime, scientific studies and medical practice have been able to demonstrate that this assumption is actually true.

The Tibetan formula *Gabur*, which is the source for the Padma Basic remedy, is used as an anti-inflammatory basic therapeutic preparation to cure "hidden fever." This refers to subliminal or chronic sources of inflammation. Medical practice has shown that Padma Basic works well with the Chinese meridian point DU-4 (Vital Gate–*Mingmen*) on the so-called "Governor Vessel."

THE POWER OF PLANT COMPONENTS

There is a long-standing relationship between plants and human beings that spans many thousands of years. Knowledgeable users have always understood how to apply the healing power of the plant world for their own benefit.

The first records of the medical use of plants are found on Sumerian clay tablets and in the Egyptian "papyrus." During their growth, plants form an abundance of bioactive substances in their flowers, leaves, and roots. These substances have an effect on the human organism when we ingest plant foods or healing herbs. Phyto-chemistry engages in a more precise study of these active substances, while pharmacology researches their therapeutic possibilities of use.

EFFECTIVENESS THROUGH DIVERSITY

Plants essentially contain two types of active substances. The products of the primary metabolism (saccharides, lipids, etc.) are indispensable for the survival of the plant itself. However, the so-called **secondary plant substances** also occur, and these can be used for healing purposes. In addition, plants provide vitamins, minerals, trace elements, antibacterial substances, and much more. The secondary phytochemicals of a plant complement and strengthen each other mutually in their effects. No isolated or chemically synthesized substances can equal this natural information structure. As in a musical composition, the perfect harmony would be lost if just one single note was missing.

There are an estimated 10,000 or more of such secondary phyto-chemicals. These serve plants as color, fragrance, and aroma substances, as well as protecting them from illnesses or pests.

Health-supporting plant substances are present in all types of grains, legumes, vegetables, and fruits, so they are already supplied to the body within the scope of a sensible diet. Although, bioactive substances exist in the food cycles only in tiny amounts, this continuous supply of minimal stimulation is what maintains many life processes.

This advantage is especially obvious in the Tibetan herbal formulas and is the actual active principle. A natural "broad-spectrum medicine" like Padma Basic can supply the organism with a variety of biochemical impulses for good health, both as a preventative measure and against existing disorders. The body is capable of filtering out precisely the information that it needs from this supply of active substances.

As in the other Tibetan plant remedies, the individual components in Padma Basic are also present in such minor amounts that Western pharmacologist would hardly expect any significant effects. Yet, this variety of gentle impulses in Padma Basic is what creates its comprehensive effect and good tolerability.

Here is a summary of some of the phyto-chemicals present in our daily food supply. It can best illustrate the extensive interaction of these natural substances.

Plant Components with **Subgroups [S]**	Found in	Actions
Essential oils and resins	spices, medicinal herbs, horseradish, mustard	usually anti-inflammatory, antiseptic, blood-purifying, immunostimulating
Bitter substances S: cynarin, lactucin, etc.	artichokes, endive, bitter herbs, etc.	digestive, calming, detoxifying
Carotinoids (precursor of vitamin A) S: beta-carotene, lycopene, etc.	yellow/orange-colored fruit and vegetables, green vegetables, tomatoes, algae, etc.	cancer prophylaxis (anticarcinogenic), antiseptic, strengthen the immune system, antioxidant (inhibits free radicals)
Tannins	roots and leaves of many plants	deprives pathogens of their breeding ground, heals wounds, soothing
Phytoestrogens S: isoflavonoids, lignans, etc.	whole grains, legumes, flaxseed, many medicinal plants	cancer prophylaxis, antiseptic, cholesterol lowering, hormone-stimulating
Phytosterols S: beta-sitosterol, etc.	plant oils and seeds, pumpkin seeds, sesame, sunflower seeds, etc.	cancer prophylaxis, cholesterol lowering
Polyphenols (see below) S: flavonoids and tannins such as anthocyanosides, quercetin, genistein, rutin, phenol acid, hydrocinnamic acid, etc.	many vegetables, red berries, onions, garlic, red grape leaves foliage, in many types of teas as green tea or rooibos tea	cancer prophylaxis, antiseptic, immune-stimulating, anti-inflammatory, regulates blood pressure, antioxidant

Cont.: Plant Components with

Subgroups [S]	Found in	Actions
Saponins (nitrogen-free glycosides)	plant seeds, legumes, many medicinal plants	cancer prophylaxis, antiseptic, cholesterol lowering, anti-inflammatory
Mucogenics	berries, many medicinal plants, such as hibiscus or Icelandic moss	soothing, protects mucous membranes
Sulphates S: ajoene, allicin, and alliin, etc.	garlic, onions and other types of plants	carcinostatic, antiseptic, stimulating, anti-inflammatory, blood-purifying, regulates digestion, antioxidant

FLAVONOIDS AND TANNINS

Among the most important plant protective substances contained in Padma Basic are the flavonoids and tannins. They have now become some of the most-researched secondary phytochemicals.

Flavonoids and tannins are subgroups of specific tannin compounds, the so-called **polyphenols.** These substances protect a plant against damage from the outside (UV radiation, fungus infection, etc.) and serve as an aid in adapting to the environment. The polyphenols have awakened the special interests of research because this substance group apparently develops a strong carcinostatic effect.

The approximately 5000 different flavonoids and tannins are primarily found in the peel and bark of fruits and vegetables, as well as in numerous tea plants and spices. They must be provided to the human organism on a regular basis since it cannot form them on its own. In the therapeutic sense, polyphenols primarily have an antioxidative effect, which means that they counteract the process of cellular aging and injury.[10] The following chapter discusses exactly how this occurs and for which health disorders the herbal mixture Padma Basic can be most useful.

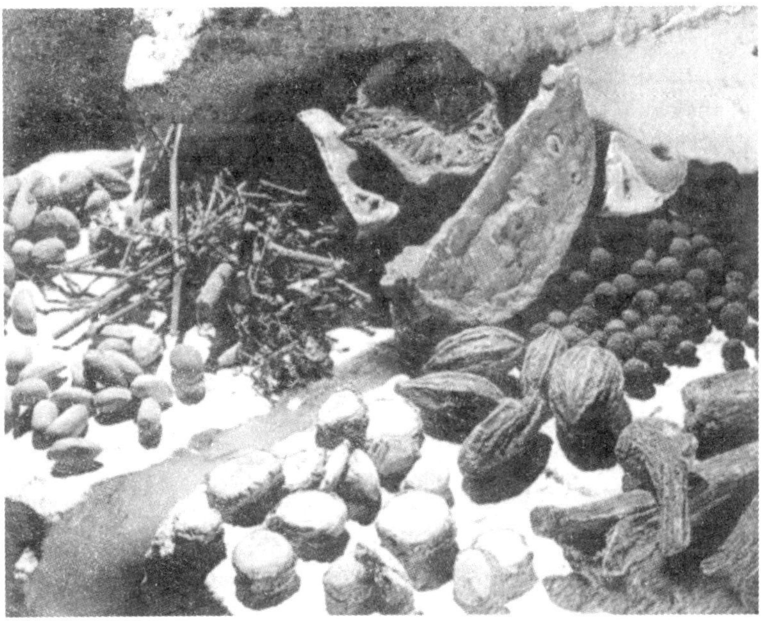

Padma Basic herbal mixture

Note: In some countries, Padma Basic additionally contains the very minor amount of 1 mg of *aconite root* (Aconiti tuber). However, as a secondary component and due to its minimal concentration it is—as Tibetan physicians have also confirmed—basically insignificant for the therapeutic effects of the remedy.

PADMA BASIC– MOTOR OF THE IMMUNE SYSTEM

Scientists have estimated that the immune system of an adult human being would weigh about 1.5 kilograms (approx. 3.3 pounds) if we were to place it on a scale. However, the employees of this biological organizational unit are distributed throughout the entire body at strategically important points. When danger threatens from the outside, which means when pathogens attempt to intrude, an initially unnoticed battle of life and death often begins. Skin and body secretions (saliva, gastric juices etc.) form an initial barrier against the enemy. If this line of defense is not successful, then the army of our immune cells is called into action.

HOW THE IMMUNE SYSTEM FUNCTIONS

The central headquarters of the **cell-linked immunity** are located in the thymus gland, which is behind the sternum. The red bone marrow serves as the producer and supply base for the immune cells, which are also present in the lymphatic system, the spleen, the tonsils and pharyngeal tonsils, the Peyer's patches of the intestines and many other organs of the body. From these collection sites, various types of white blood corpuscles (leucocytes) are sent into the field a battle troops against intruding bacteria, viruses, and fungi. Their main task consists of defending against foreign microorganisms with the help of enzymes, protective substances and by means of **phagocytosis** (which causes particulate material to be ingested by cells).

Of the cells formed in the bone marrow, 70% are granulocytes (phagocytes with a grainy appearance); the rest of those formed are monocytes (giant phagocytes or macrophages), as well as lymphocytes, which can produce antibodies (see below). In addition to the cell-linked portion, there is also a **humoral part of the immune system**, which is associated with the blood and the lymph. This also keeps a constant watch for foreign bodies. Its task is the production of antibodies or immunoglobuline through the **B lymphocytes**, while the main protagonists of the cell-mediated defense are the **T lymphocytes** and T helper cells.

ANTIBODIES AND ANTIGENS

In a healthy organism, every infection immediately triggers a humoral or a cell-controlled immune response. Undesired intruders are initially recognized as exogenous protein **(antigen)**. B and T cells then react with the formation of antibodies. We could say that they mark the enemy in order to hand it over to the special killer cells and phagocytes destruction. Afterward, some of the lymphocytes assume the function of memory cells. They virtually store the blueprint of the undesired guests. If this occurs again, then the recognition of the enemy and the formation of antibodies take place much more quickly and efficiently. In such cases, we are "immune."

Consequently, every human being possesses a series of innate and acquired defense mechanisms against infections. The biological correlations of this complex regulation cycle have by no means been adequately researched.

But this much is certain: Only a well-functioning immune system can effectively protect us against damage to our health. Today it must deal with an extreme number of irritations and burdens.

Above all, a decrease in the powers of the immune system through environmental toxins, misuse of medications and substances such as tobacco, alcohol, and caffeine, improper diet, lack of exercise, and psychological problems. Many ailments, especially those of a chronic nature, can only spread through the body when the immune system has been compromised by health disorders that have not been properly healed or a long-term harmful lifestyle. In the Western world, this applies in particular to the so-called diseases of modern civilization: cardiovascular diseases, cancer, and premature degenerative processes such as those that we generally interpret to be "symptoms of old age."

KILLER CELLS AND CONTROL CELLS– HARMONY IS EVERYTHING

An intact immune system is in a state of dynamic equilibrium. With each "attack of the enemy," this equilibrium is shifted in the direction of humoral or cell-dependent activity and must therefore adjust itself each time anew. The cell-controlled defense accomplishes a large portion of its defense work with the help of the T lymphocytes. A subspecies of these immune cells fights in form of **killer cells** against attackers from the outside; when they have completed their work, they are slowed down by another group, the **suppressor or control cells.**

However, when the relationship between killer and control cells is no longer balanced, the immunological equilibrium is disturbed. If too many killer cells are at work and the control cells do not succeed in stopping their desire to attack, then their attacks begin to be directed against the body itself. In plain English: Our defense police wrongly recognize the body's own cell tissue as foreign and try to destroy it. Such dysfunctions are also called **autoimmune diseases** and are a major cause for complaints such as the rheumatic diseases, many allergies including asthma, multiple sclerosis (destruction of the nerves of the brain and spinal cord), lupus erythematosus, myasthenia gravis (chronic muscle weakness), to leukemia. But inner organs (thyroid gland, adrenal glands, etc.) can also be affected.

In the opposite case, the control cells do their task too well and prevent the killer cells, which are usually already weakened, from doing their job. The result is a far-reaching failure of the body's defenses, which encourages the development of chronic diseases. Infections are then free to spread without any obstacles. An extreme example of the complete collapse of all immune responses can be seen in the AIDS syndrome. Since medical research has began discovering these correlations, the necessity for gentle therapies without side effects that do not additionally weaken and impair the defense system has been even more pronounced.

STRESS AND FREE RADICALS

During the 1950s, Dr. Denham Harman, a professor at the University of Nebraska College of Medicine, presented a revolutionary thesis: the theory of aging through free radicals. It stated that illness and cell deterioration occur when our body cells are permanently damaged through the attacks by so-called free radicals.[11]

Although little attention was given to it at first, Harman's theory serves as the foundation for further research on the development of modern diseases, including the problems of cancer and AIDS.

But what is a free radical?

In addition to energy, each body cell also requires oxygen (Latin: *oxygenium)* for its metabolism. It is supplied with it through the respiration and the blood circulation. The oxidation (burning of oxygen) that occurs during this process is the foundation of all higher life forms. But our cell metabolism continuously also produces harmful by-products—and these are the free radicals. This occurs in the following manner: Molecules usually consist of one atomic nucleus, as well as a pair of electrons. On the other hand, free radicals are unstable, highly reactive oxygen molecules that are missing an electron in their chemical structure. These "unfinished" molecules can trigger fatal chain reactions. Namely, they attempt to tear foreign electrons out of healthy cellular bonds, which causes the development of toxic compounds. Free radicals react in an especially lively manner with unsaturated residues of fatty acids. As a result, new aggressive molecular debris is continuously formed. This process can only be stopped by specific **"radical-scavengers"** (see below).

In this way, millions of tiny individual damages occur within our cells every day, accelerating their aging process. These can be the triggers for cell degeneration (cancer and other tumors, DNA damage, etc.). This means that our bodies are constantly exposed to bombardment from both inside and outside (through environmental toxins, food, UV radiation, ground-level ozone, etc.). They weaken the immune system and are the concomitant causes of the above-mentioned modern disorders. The general term used for this battle situation that our organism must continuously master is **oxidative stress**. This reason alone suffices to make the theory of free radicals a crucial point in the search for the ultimate causes of disease, aging, and death.

THE ROLE OF ANTIOXIDANTS

In order to control the raging of the free radicals, nature—and therefore the human body—has developed effective weapons: the antioxidants.

The largest part of this work is performed by the body's own enzymes. They are capable of stopping free radicals by providing them with the missing electrons and thereby transform them into harmless products of decay. In addition, we can effectively support the continual "clean-up campaign" of the body through a regular supply of natural antioxidants from plant foods.

Among the substances with a strong antioxidant effect, as we now know, are beta-carotene (provitamin A), vitamins C and E, the trace elements zinc and selenium, glutathione, lipoic acid, as well as the vitamin-like coenzyme Q-10. But there are probably many other biochemicals that in some way have an antioxidative effect. However, the therapeutic effect of high dosage synthetic preparations is rightfully doubted. These substances are namely most effective when we take them in their original form of natural, high-quality foods, spice herbs, and medicinal plants.

The multi-substance combination **Padma Basic** contains an abundance of antioxidant, immune-stimulating substances that perfectly complement and strengthen each other in their harmonious interplay.

BIOPHOTONS– GLOWING EGGS AND HAPPY CHICKENS

Antioxidants never carried out their functions in isolation from each other. There is "teamwork" everywhere in nature, and the cells of the immune systems also can only fulfill their tasks only when it is possible for them to communicate with each other. But how does this occur?

NO LIFE WITHOUT LIGHT

It is no coincidence that the Biblical sentence "let there be light" symbolizes the beginning of all life. In fact, extremely weak light signals radiate from the living organisms of the cell nuclei. The smallest energy building blocks of light are called light quantums or photons. When the German quantum physicist Fritz A. Popp began to study these tiny light particles many decades ago, he coined the expression **biophotons** (ultraweak photon emission from biological systems) to describe them.

This cell radiation, also called luminescence when it is ultra weak, has controlling functions within the organism. Our body's defense works with such light signals. Immune cells can apparently communicate with each other in this way, exchanging important messages and information.

The biophoton research has provided many fascinating findings. At times its experiments have been beneficial to the modern food industry and prove that the protection of animals also means the protection of human beings. This statement applies to the simple chicken egg. Comparisons namely show that organic eggs from "happy" free-range chickens "glow" much more strongly than those from fowl that must eke out their poor, short lives in tight cage batteries.[12] Anyone who still doubts the better digestibility of free-range eggs is probably beyond help. But how is all of this related to Padma Basic?

PADMA–STRENGTHENED CELLS SHINE BRIGHTER

Every continuing immunological stress in the body is accompanied by inflammatory reactions. In this process, the phagocytes and macrophages attend to the elimination of occurring cell debris and maintain the inflammation as long as necessary in order to remove the waste from the body through such substances as pus and wound secretions. Free radicals are also formed during this process of debridement. But they are not initially capable of doing any harm because the entire process takes place within the phagocytes.

After the successful "digestion of the enemy," inflammatory reaction also subsides—or it should at least.

If the immune system is supported in such situations through the ingestion of Padma Basic, a distinctly strengthened radiation of light from the immune cells can observed; moreover, the components of this medicine formula are apparently also capable of once again subduing the inflammatory reaction after a successful defense.

When there is a chronic inflammation, the phagocytes remain constantly activated. Then they begin to release the free radicals to the surrounding tissue and damage healthy cell structures. In this case, the effect of Padma Basic consists of a specific regulation and subduing of the immune response. The over-stimulated organism is then gently but firmly brought back into order. Among other things, the components of Padma Basic inhibit the activity of the enzyme elastase, a protein-splitting substance that is considerably involved in the destruction of tissue through chronic sites of inflammation. The abundance of natural antioxidants with a polyphenol character (flavonoids and tannins) permits the chronic inflammations to heal more easily since the body is offered numerous impulses for self-regulation.[13]

CLINICAL APPLICATIONS OF PADMA BASIC

Comparative studies have proved that a causative correlation with oxidative stress can be suspected for more than 100 different syndromes. These include asthmatic ailments in which inflammatory cells are found in the lung area, as well as chronic-inflammatory intestinal diseases (colitis ulcerosa, Crohn's disease), the dangerous plaques in arteriosclerotic vessels or diabetes mellitus.

As the **biochemist Marianne Suter** from the ETH, the *Swiss Federal Institute of Technology* in Zurich, explains that Padma Basic can release electrons, which means it also has a reductive effect on free radicals. She was able to demonstrate this by means of an analytic system in which a specific protein by the name of "cytochrome C" was used. In this experiment, Padma Basic was able to reduce the harmful cytochrome C and thereby ensure effective protection of the cells.[14]

Even in small doses, *Padma Basic*'s ability to neutralize free radicals is at least as strong as those of the antioxidants vitamins C, E, and beta-carotene. This herbal formula may therefore be extremely effective in subduing excessive immune reactions, which are a symptom of so-called autoimmune diseases (see above). According to the current standard of knowledge, the long-term ingestion of Padma Basic therefore appears to be highly recommended for all forms of immune weakness and susceptibility to infections.[15]

The Hamburg physician, author and Tibet expert Dr. Egbert Asshauer reported on the application of Padma Basic for his patient after an outbreak of the AIDS infection. As a result, it was possible to keep this man's blood levels stable and considerably increase his quality of life.[16] Here is an interesting fact in relation to this disease: In a Tibetan medicine book of the 13th Century, a syndrome was described that practically mirrors the symptoms of AIDS. In any case, the therapy-accompanying administration of Padma Basic should also be advantageous for HIV-positive patients in strengthening their immune functions.[17]

However, it is appropriate to make an important statement here to those who want to use Padma Basic to improve their health: Never stop taking prescribed medications on your own; only do this with the approval of your physician/naturopath. He or she will help you determine the most appreciate approach for you. However, also do not let yourself be intimidated if you encounter ignorance and rejection. According to the current state of knowledge, Padma Basic does not have a negative influence on any other therapy, while it probably can considerably improve your general state of health.

A MEDICINE AGAINST AGING?

Oxidative long-term causes an over-activation and ultimately a weakening of the thymus, which then continuously produces less and less T cells. The thymus gland is considered the "life clock" of the organism. With increasing age, this organ begins to shrink. The waning of its functions leads to death.

Our hopes of discovering a "fountain of youth" is legendary—and this is also what it will remain since the aging process is genetically preprogrammed (and we would be wise to not force the disruption of this program). The genetic code is inscribed within every cell of the body. It controls all of the cell functions from birth and growth up until the occurrence of death. With advancing age, this source of information begins to become less reliable. The situation is similar to that of a construction site where the contractor is increasingly less capable of giving the correct instructions to the army of his workers. The first dysfunctions begin to occur. In relation to aging, we speak quite aptly about "manifestations of old age": wrinkling of the skin, attrition of the bones and joints, vascular sclerosis (arteriosclerosis), loss of vigor, weakening of the intellectual abilities (senility), and so forth.

Geriatric researchers have long known that cell damage caused by oxidation, meaning the havoc created by the free radicals, also plays a significant role here. Probably the worst example of rapid cell aging is progeria, a shocking syndrome in which children already assume the appearance of old people with all signs of approaching death. Well-known degenerative ailments like Parkinson's or Alzheimer's disease also appear to be the result of harmful oxidation processes in the cells.

SPECIFIC FOOD SUPPLEMENTATION AS A SOLUTION

Generations before us already knew that a varied, natural diet keeps people young and healthy. However, the decisive role that our immune system plays in this has only recently been clearly acknowledged by science.

In many test series, giving human beings with ailments caused by the aging process a well-balanced supply of vitamins, minerals, and trace elements led to a conspicuous improvement of their condition. In many cases, it was possible to stop mental symptoms of deterioration and improve the defense against infections. The scientific facts that are available about Padma Basic on the whole permit the conclusion that the antioxidant natural substances that it contains—especially the polyphenols—are suitable for favorably influencing deterioration due to the aging process and possibly even delaying them under certain circumstances. Because of its immune-strengthening effect, Padma Basic therefore represents a meaningful preparation for maintaining the physical and mental functions as a supplement to our daily food intake.

Our diet should naturally also be oriented toward unprocessed, high-quality food: fruit, vegetables, whole-grain products, seeds, nuts and kernels, occasionally fish; milk products and eggs in moderation, and very little meat and sweets. Adequate exercise provides the body with oxygen and creates the absolutely necessary balance required for the prevention of the problems related to stress.

AN IMPORTANT NOTE

Under the key words of "supporting the immune systems," it is important to mention that Padma Basic should also be a good remedy for avoiding the increasingly frequent occurrence of complications after vaccinations. Without wanting to judge the value of this preventive measure, we should remember that especially children suffer from fever, gastrointestinal disorders, skin rashes, or even worse problems after being vaccinated. These problems are probably a result of the increasingly weakened or even untrained immune system that reacts excessively to the irritations. Undetected allergies often occur in response to the additives and preservatives contained in the vaccine.

Since Padma Basic can already be given to small children (mixed with fruit sauce or porridge), this could be a significant possibility for giving the irritated immune system additional assistance in mastering such an acute irritation therapy.

PADMA BASIC AND ARTERIOSCLEROSIS

Let me introduce this chapter with a story that is repeated thousands of times every day: Mr. X, a man in his fifties who is a heavy smoker and not opposed to taking extra helpings of a tasty meal, suddenly begins to feel tingling in his legs. The circulation in the lower extremities is not as good as it should be. The distances that this man, who was previously quite agile, can walk without pain become shorter and shorter—a major handicap in his occupation as a craftsman.

It is naturally time for him to now radically change his diet and general lifestyle habits, which his physician urgently advises him to do. But we all know from personal experience how difficult this actually is in the practice. Mr. X hopes that the appropriate medications will help his body get back into shape. He thinks he is not capable of changing his lifestyle. So the inevitable happens: The ailment increasingly worsens. The amputation of a leg can no longer be avoided. This is followed by several heart attacks and ultimately a long, torturous lingering illness. None of the medical arts are effective against the irreparable vascular damage that has occurred through the decades.

This tragic story could also have happened, for example, to Ms. Y, a professionally and personally successful woman in her late forties, who at times complains about "too much stress." She would have been very typical of our Western "power society" in which the female sex is quickly catching up in terms of cardiovascular disease. The overall lifestyle and behavior plays a decisive role here, something that both Mr. X and Ms. Y were aware of. But, despite the many "sins," are there still perhaps ways of repairing some of the damage? Would something like Tibetan medicine with its plant remedies be an opportunity that still offers some support when all of the other paths are already closed? And what does it offer in terms of prevention?

A SCOURGE OF HUMANITY

Statistics make it clear: During the course of the 20th Century, cardiovascular diseases in the Western nations has turned into the Number One cause of death.

The second place is occupied by cancer diseases and third is held by another malady typical of modern civilization: stroke (CVA). Around the globe, according to the World Health Organization (WHO), more than one billion human beings were the victims of heart attacks or strokes during the last 100 hundred years. In the industrial nations, we must reckon with one person dying from a heart attack every second. However, we would hardly expect the following fact to be true: The main cause of this misery, arteriosclerosis, which is also called "hardening of the arteries" by the general public, and all of its consecutive symptoms, is not at all a modern disease of affluent society; to the contrary, it is a very ancient one.

If we take a brief look at the era around 2,000 B.C.: Under Pharaoh Ramses II, the advanced Egyptian civilization once again achieved an unimagined blossoming. Many centuries later, the French physician and Egyptologist Sir Marc Armand Ruffer found severe arteriosclerotic vessel changes in this royal mummy. This was not a surprise since the God-King Ramses died at a very old age. However, the tissue incisions from other mummies showed that vascular damage and metabolic ailments (for example, gout) were no less widespread at that time than they are today.

Coincidence? Hardly.

At least the members of the upper class had no limitations placed upon them in terms of what they ate. The well-situated average Egyptian of those times was certainly much more corpulent than the embellished relief depictions would have us believe. Purulent infections of the teeth and tonsils occurred frequently and encouraged the development of angiopathy. On the other hand, the regular distribution of garlic rations together with a simple diet largely protected the Egyptian working class against the malady of arteriosclerosis.

As we know, garlic has the effect of protecting the arteries. Especially in recent time, increasingly more experts are postulating that sclerotic vessels are primarily the result of long-term improper diets and nutritional deficiencies. The adequate supply of specific vitamins and other biochemicals is a factor that has certainly been given too little attention in relation to arteriosclerosis.

DEVELOPMENT AND RISK FACTORS OF ARTERIAL OCCLUSIVE DISEASES

Circulatory disorders are the most frequently discussed topic in the health press. Every normal person now knows that an unhealthy lifestyle has negative effects on the elasticity and functionality of our vessels. The blood-vessel system provides the body with oxygen and nutrients.

When its functional capacity diminishes, we immediately feel it.

WHAT IS ARTERIOSCLEROSIS?

Commonly called "hardening of the arteries," arteriosclerosis (also: arterial sclerosis) occurs through damage to the walls of the blood-conducting arterial vessels. A fatty diet, for example, reduces the blood's ability to flow and leads to a greater possibility of coagulation. On the smooth inner skin (tunica intima) of the arteries, fatty substances are deposited; these, in turn, obstruct the bloodstream. The result is a chronic-inflammatory process that can end with the complete obstruction of a vessel. In addition, the arteries lose their natural elasticity through the calcific deposits and turn into stiff pipes.

Experience has shown that the first symptoms occur when more than half of the vascular lumen is closed—and then also only if there is physical strain. According to where in the body this process takes place, the consequences range from painful arms and legs that "fall asleep" to the life-threatening heart attack as a result of the occlusion of fine coronary vessels. The blood clots or tissue particles (emboli) deposited on the walls of the arteries can also be washed away and abruptly interrupt the oxygen supply to distant parts of the body. Embolism of the inner organs and/or strokes in the brain can then occur. For those affected by this malady, it is important to understand that these dramatic functional disorders are just the final point in a process that has gone on for decades. Consequently, this is a development that can be prevented and its risk factors can be largely eliminated.

SCARCITY IN ABUNDANCE

What causes arteriosclerosis to develop is still a topic of debate. There is solely agreement on the fact that the "concentration" of several circumstances that have been recognized as dangerous drastically increases the probability of suffering damage to the vessel walls.

The following risk factors have been determined as causes for arteriosclerosis: unhealthy lifestyle (smoking, alcohol, a fatty diet, lack of exercise), environmental pollution (above all, heavy metals), long-term psychological stress ("the manager disease"), as well as certain hereditary tendencies toward vascular damage. The triggering factor of high blood pressure is today seen in the larger correlation. It is part of the so-called **"metabolic syndrome"**.

This clinical picture characterizes the well-fed average citizen of our high-performance society. Renunciation and moderation are very difficult for him. His knowledge about a healthy diet is inadequate or he ignores it. He does not participate enough in sports and exercise. He pays for this with overweight, diabetes, elevated blood lipids (LDL cholesterol and triglycerides), and uric-acid levels. The lapse of the metabolic functions is now just a matter of time. High blood pressure and vascular occlusions are the predictable consequences.

Quite recently, a "new" risk factor has been discovered: **homocysteine (Hcy).** Homocysteine is an intermediate metabolic product that occurs when the body utilizes the vital amino acid methionine. At an excessive concentration, this can damage the walls of the arteries. But if we now label this Hcy as the culprit in general, this would be just as short-sighted as the attempt to treat arteriosclerosis solely by lowering the blood cholesterol. In contrast with this approach, too little attention has been given to the possibilities of nutrition therapy. Elevated levels of homocysteine can, as we now also know, actually be lowered through the adequate intake of the vitamins B6, B12, TMG and especially folic acid. But this is hardly the complete solution to the mystery. Nature just doesn't function in such a simple way.

MODERN THERAPY APPROACHES

As much as we may be aware of certain errors in the way we live our lives, we often only think of correcting them when all of the alarms are ringing.

This is one more reason for modern medicine to concentrate on the therapy of existing vascular damage. In part, it is very successful in doing this, as shown in the rapid development of heart surgery. Foreign hearts are transplanted, constricted vessels are expanded, and bypasses are created. Gene technology now even makes it possible to grow new blood vessels. But is this really the most meaningful way to deal with the miracle of the human body? Shouldn't our attention be directed instead to the gentle methods of prevention and therapy that have no side effects?

CELLULAR MEDICINE– A NEW UNDERSTANDING OF HEALTH

Health and illness take place on the cellular level, and this fact has been known for many years. If these are not given proper nutrition, meaning that they are not supplied with all of the important biochemicals, problems arise. Why should this situation be different for arteriosclerosis?

The suppositions that an inadequate supply of vitamins, minerals, and other biological substances are the main causes for inflammatory focal manifestations in blood vessels are by no means random. Studies have proven that specific doses of vitamin E lower the risk of heart attack by more than 40%. Vitamin C has been identified as effective vascular protection since, among other things, it promotes the break-down of cholesterol. On the other hand, a lack of vitamin C encourages the development of lesions in the vessel wall and therefore the formation of sclerotic deposits. But if the use of synthetic vitamins achieves such a high rate of success, imagine how much better a composition of natural, synergistic (mutually strengthening) natural substances must work.

A formidable indication of how powerful nature can be in healing is the traditional use of garlic as a remedy against "hardening of the arteries" and age-related complaints. Although this idea was long ridiculed by modern science, we know today that its components actually have a prophylactic effect and can very well stop the advancement of arteriosclerosis.

IS ARTERIOSCLEROSIS CURABLE?

In 1990, the *Lancet*, an internationally recognized medical journal, attracted a great deal of attention when it published the latest research findings from California. Physicians had succeeded in proving that a correction of lifestyle leads to the regression of sclerotic vascular changes. Even after just one year, the coronary sclerosis (narrowing of the coronary vessels) that had been diagnosed in the test subjects showed distinct improvement without any type of medications. Up to this time, the possibility of such a regression had generally been doubted.

This study, called **The Life Style Heart Trial**, along with other publications, had emphatically shown how arteriosclerosis can be outwitted through a modified diet and change in lifestyle (exercise, relaxation techniques, etc.). In the area of nutritional therapy, it seems appropriate to give the body specific biological information, in addition to high-quality foods, that help it remain its equilibrium. This task can be fulfilled in an ideal manner by complex Tibetan herbal mixtures such as Padma Basic. They give the organism gentle, but continuous orientation help in activating its natural powers of self-healing.

PADMA BASIC AS AN EFFECTIVE THERAPEUTIC AGENT

When Karl Lutz, the "discoverer" of Padma Basic, had the first Tibetan formulas made with the help of his newly established Swiss herbal company, he could not have imagined that the Number 28 in particular of his "Padma" series would acquire such an astonishing reputation. He gave the Tibetan medicines, together with a list of indications, to some of the physicians he visited on a regular basis as a pharmaceutical salesman.

In 1966, Dr. Charles, M.D. in the Swiss city of Winterthur prescribed the formula No. 28 for one of his patients. He was the municipal president of the neighboring town and suffered from an advanced case of arterial occlusion in his legs. Medications had shown no satisfactory effects, but after taking Padma Basic for a number of weeks, this man could ultimately once again walk several kilometers without pain, which had been unthinkable before. This case caused quite a sensation.

Encouraged by this success, Dr. Charles gave Padma Basic to other patients with arteriosclerosis, who also soon showed improvement. Subsequent studies at the Zurich University Clinic confirmed this little wonder. The professional world began to sit up and take notice.[18]

HELP FOR THE SMOKERS' LEG

Smoking is an undisputed risk factor for arteriosclerosis.

Nicotine elevates the fibrinogen level in the blood, meaning that it promotes its coagulation. The danger of vascular occlusions through blood clots is distinctly increased, advancing an existing case of arteriosclerosis. In this situation, pain frequently occurs because of the circulation disorders in the lower extremities: the so-called smokers' leg. The patient is hardly capable of walking longer distances without pain and must frequently take a break. Medical terminology calls this clinical picture intermittent claudication (Latin: *claudicatio intermittens).*

In 1977, the first double-blind study with Padma Basic was conducted on patients with peripheral arterial occlusion disease (PAOD) of the legs at the *Lucerne Canton Hospital.* (Double-blind study means that neither the physician nor the patients know which participants are receiving the medication that is being tested and which ones are receiving placebo, a substance without any effective components, during the experiment.) The distances that they were able to walk without pain increased by 54% for the test subjects treated with Padma Basic. On the other hand, the vasodilating agents of conventional medicine, the so-called vasodilators, only achieved a maximum increase of 10%. In addition, Padma Basic did not show the strong side effects that these medications generally have.[19]

A large-scale double-blind experiment on 43 patients in 1985 proved that there was quite a considerable increase in the maximum distance that those taking Padma Basic could walk without pain in comparison to the untreated persons. The participants whose condition had significantly improved were treated daily with 3 times 2 capsules of Padma Basic for 16 weeks.

In 1998, a new pilot study showed that Padma Basic distinctly promotes the normalization of the systolic blood pressure at the ankle after strenuous walking exercise.[20]

In the meantime, Padma Basic is now one of the best-studied natural remedies in the world. It has proved to have excellent tolerability and practically no side effects.

HOW PADMA BASIC WORKS

A team of researchers working with Dr. Kaj Winter from the University of Copenhagen attempted, in what has probably been the most substantial study with patients suffering from smokers' leg, to clarify the question of how Padma Basic influences arterial vascular occlusions. Laboratory tests showed that Padma Basic shortens the time required for dissolving blood clots in the legs because it inhibits the endogenic (body's own) substances that prevent this dissolution. As prophylaxis, Padma Basic contributes to a lowering of the blood lipids (triglycerides and LDL cholesterol) and makes it more difficult for the fatty substances to be deposited on the vessel wall. Its effect is additionally improved so that it also alleviates inflammatory reactions, as described in the previous chapter.[21]

In no case should we give in to the illusion that Padma Basic is a "remedy" for existing cases of arteriosclerosis since it only influences it indirectly, which means that it cannot eliminate it. However, it is known that when there are vascular occlusions the body attempts to activate a replacement system, the so-called collateral arterial bypass system. During this phase of reestablishing blood flow, it is already possible for life-threatening disorders to occur. Padma Basic apparently helps in accelerating this process of readjustment.

According to the Tibetan approach, the energy of Wind, which is stimulated by Padma Basic, is related to the blood-vessel system of the heart, among other things. So it is no coincidence that patients with coronary circulation disorders report of an improvement of their complaints (chest pain, shortness of breath). Some of them even claim that Padma Basic saved their lives (see the chapter "Case Histories—This Is How Padma Basic Helped Me"). This statement cannot be contradicted since there is at least one double-blind study on the application of Padma Basic in cases of angina pectoris.[22]

Although there is no longer any doubt about the value of Padma Basic as an effective therapeutic agent, its greatest strength lies in the area of prevention. People who are at risk for arteriosclerosis are advised to pay attention even at the first signs of circulatory disorders such as tingling, formication, the feeling that the hands and feet are falling asleep, or muscle cramps in the calves. At the same time, these individuals should attempt to correct their life style and eating habits, stop smoking, and reduce any excess weight. If they additionally supplement their diet by taking Padma Basic as a "bio-regulator," this approach should soon show positive results. The difference will naturally not be felt immediately, especially if there are no significant complaints. However, the benefit of this "readjustment" for the body is shown at latest when individuals can master everyday life in a more active and healthy manner than before, when their metabolic levels (once again) register in the normal range, and when arteriosclerosis is no longer a nightmare for them.

Those who are already suffering from serious disorders of the arterial circulation should only take Padma Basic in addition to the prescribed therapy and inform their physician of this. As soon as tangible improvement is noted, the physician can then adjust the medication accordingly. In their own interests, patients should never do this on their own.

PRACTICAL EXPERIENCES CONFIRM EXTENSIVE ACTIVE PROFILE

According to an evaluated, comprehensive practice study from 2001, Padma Basic may do much more than just stimulate the peripheral circulation. Through its synergistic effects, it also positively influences an entire series of complaints, most of which occur as a result of a poor blood supply.

HIGHLY EFFECTIVE AND WELL TOLERATED

The above-mentioned study is based on a total of 147 empiric reports from 15 Swiss physicians, including 9 gener al practitioners, 3 surgeons, and 1 specialist for leg disorders, 1 internist, and 1 dentist.

In 60% of the cases, Padma Basic was used as the main medication for peripheral circulatory disorders; 94% of the participants showed improvement as a result. About half of the patients showing improvement took no other medication besides Padma Basic. The tolerability was evaluated as very good and side-effects (stomach complaints) were minimal at a rate of only 4%. For the cardiovascular diseases (angina pectoris, etc.), 12 of the 13 cases improved (with accompanying medication).

However, the remarkable thing about this study was that many patients were additionally able to observe a remission of memory problems and vision disorders. These complaints often accompany circulation disorders of the head region. At the same time, there was a distinctly positive change in the afflicted emotional state of some of the test participants (see pages 77ff.).

Moreover, it is very interesting that 3 of the 4 study participants with **tinnitus** (ringing in the ears) showed a significant improvement in the complaints, 2 of them without any other type of therapy. One patient was completely cured of intensive tinnitus after 6 months. A participant with **Meniere's disease** (vertigo of the inner ear) was free of complaints after 5 months (accompanying hypotensive medication). In all of these cases, the dosage was: 3 times 2 tablets of Padma Basic daily.

A patient with type II diabetes (late-onset diabetes) discovered a reduction of the levels, which could at least partly be contributed to the ingestion of Padma Basic (more about diabetes in the chapter on "Case Histories—This Is How Padma Basic Helped Me").

PADMA BASIC CAN DO EVEN MORE

In addition to relieving complaints that are clearly based on an insufficient blood supply, the above study was able to prove that Padma

Basic has a beneficial influence on an entire series of additional syndromes because of its harmonizing properties. The mutual characteristic of these ailments is oxidative stress and a dysfunction of the immune system.

There were also improvements of severe to weak symptoms, and even an elimination of the complaints, in cases of:

- Hypercholesterolemia (with accompanying diet, but without lipid-lowering agents)
- Back ailments/pain in the joints (arthrosis, sciatica, carpal-tunnel syndrome)
- Allergies (pollen allergy, asthma, dermatoses)
- Weakness, tiredness, and dizziness (without additional medications)
- Chronic bronchitis, sinusitis, pulmonary emphysema
- Vascular disorders
- Migraines with auras (seeing bright lights)
- Parkinson's disease

The dentist who participated in this study used Padma Basic to support the elimination of heavy metals when removing amalgam and for better healing of wounds.

PADMA BASIC AND CANCER

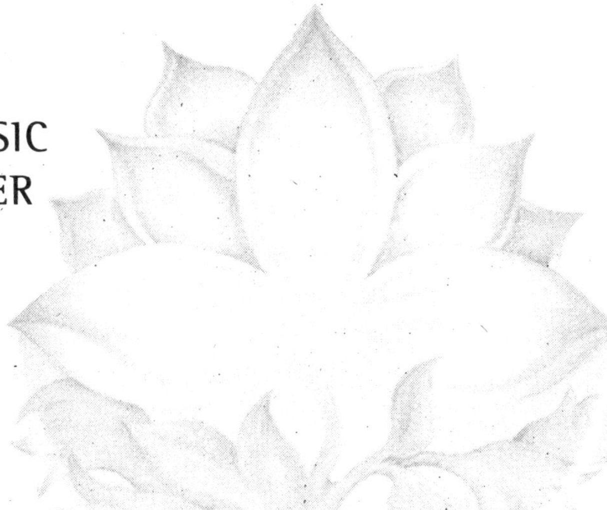

Writing about cancer is always a delicate matter, as every author knows. This chapter is intended to offer an insight into current research and therapy, as well as explaining the diverse backgrounds. However, it is not my intention to polarize or awaken false hopes. To come straight to the point: Padma Basic is obviously not a "remedy" against cancer, but it may, as described in the following, be able to produce certain results.

CANCER– PANDEMONIUM IN THE CELLULAR STATE

Cancer is the name of a malignant new growth of cells. The Latin word "cancer" is based on the idea that the physicians of Ancient Greece believed each cancer tumor develops venous networks in the form of crab feet. Even long before two German scientists discovered the cells almost at the same time in the 19th Century, cancerous proliferations were not something unknown. Cancer has always afflicted humanity, and it occurs in every corner of the world. Despite all of the factors that we today know increase the risk of developing cancer, this disease has a great multitude of causes, some of which are still unknown. Yet, we now know one thing for sure: Cancer is related to cell aging.

In earlier times, when the average life expectancy was very limited, most human beings in the northern latitudes simply did not live long enough to experience cancer. Cancer is largely a consequence of the (biological) aging of our cells. As a result, the cellular condition of even very young human beings can already fall into the category of "old" when there is an accumulation of risk factors. The fateful role that the free radicals play in this process has already been explained. So this once again brings us back to the immune system because our body defense ultimately decides every battle for life and death.

CANCER CELLS ARE CLEVER

The first medical professional to emphatically point out a correlation between curing cancer and the immune system was the American surgeon Dr. William B. Coley. To his amazement, he discovered that a tumor patient who had successfully survived a major bacterial infection also showed no more evidence of the cancer tumor. Apparently, the illness of the man activated his defense system and made it capable of also recognizing and defeating the cancer. Afterward, Coley attempted to manufacture a vaccine for cancer patients; however, this attempt was not successful.[23]

So what makes it so difficult for our immune system to recognize degenerated cells? How do cancer occur and develop in the first place? To discover an answer to this, we must first look at normal cell growth: Billions of body cells die every day and must be replaced through division. Each time this occurs, two new identical cells are created. Specific protein substances ensure the correct flow of information as a type of safety switch. If something goes wrong, the respective cell receives the command to self-destruct. However, sometimes (and this occurs with increasing frequency at an advanced age) some cells succeed in slipping through this security net. They begin a process of uncontrolled division. In medical terms, these are then considered to be cancerous.

DISGUISING AND DECEIVING

Just like every intruder from the outside, cancer cells also have an antigen on their membrane that allows the killer cells of our immune systems to recognize them as foreign bodies. An intact defense is almost always the victor in this case and renders the "criminals in the cellular state" harmless. However, this is the fatal thing about tumor cells: Some of them know how to remove the telltale "marker" and therefore escape unscathed. B and T lymphocytes can no longer recognize them as the enemy. Furthermore, the cancer cell is capable of coating its outer wall with a thick layer of fibrin that covers the marking antigen. Each cell possesses this fibrin layer, but it is formed up to 15 times as thick in cancer tissue. In addition, fibrin serves as a type of adhesive substance for conglomerating cells, which allows the tumor to continually grow. Cancer cells can hardly be surpassed in terms of cleverness and insidiousness.

After it reaches a certain size, the cancer tumor also finds a possibility of signaling the surrounding blood vessels to nourish it. This process is called **angiogenesis**, and this is how new blood capillaries are created to supply the tumor with nutritive substances and pave the way for a proliferation of new cancer cells (metastasis) throughout the entire body. Very few patients actually die because of the initial tumor; on the contrary, it is the metastases that attack the vital organs and destroy them. How Tibetan multi-substance mixtures can intervene in a helpful manner will be described further below.

CANCER AS A SYSTEMIC DISEASE

Cancer research (oncology) works throughout the world with all its power to develop new remedies and better diagnostic possibilities. We often hear that more facts are required. However, this much is true: We have an excess of facts but apparently cannot translate them into action effectively enough. It appears clear that cancer is not a localized occurrence; instead, it has the character of a chronic systemic disease.

Although an operation may eliminate the primary tumor, we do not know when and where the system will degenerate and produce more cancer cells. Conventional medicine attempts to cope with its proliferation through hormones, radiation therapy, and chemotherapy. These are methods that—although they have been greatly improved in the meantime—are usually associated with strong side-effects and frequently prove to be inadequate in helping the patient. We also know this: Every cancerous disease occurs in episodes. It is not unusual for metastases to appear shortly after surgical operations. One reason for this is certainly the lasting strain and weakening of the immune systems, which is why every cancer patient should endeavor to rebuild and strengthen it. On the one hand, this includes avoiding the well-known risk factors (smoking, alcohol, environmental toxins, extreme exposure to the sun, etc.); on the other hand, a natural lifestyle and diet must be observed, as already has been discussed in the chapter on arteriosclerosis. The immune system can be effectively supported and promoted in its functions by a Tibetan multi-substance medicine such as **Padma Basic.**

PREVENTION AND TREATMENT

Our modern prevention program (which everyone should use, in any case) can hardly disguise this fact: The so-called early cancer diagnosis is actually a late diagnosis. A visible cancer tumor in the size of a pea already has more than around 200 (!) million cells and has developed completely without symptoms on the average over a time period of eight to ten years. Once again, this illustrates how important it is to take preventive action while we are still healthy.

THE LIVER AS THE HEALTH GUARDIAN

Even if students at the universities hear very little about it and most physicians neglect it as a result: The liver is the most important organ of all for our health. This is simple to understand when we take a closer look at its range of functions.

As the **central detoxification organ,** this approximately 1.5 kilogram heavy gland plays a key role in the organism. The liver is a perfect chemical factory. It purifies our blood of harmful substances, produces bile for digestion, and regulates the sugar and fat metabolism, as well as our body heat. Furthermore, it provides for the formation of red blood corpuscles, which supply our cells with oxygen. (An oxygen deficiency in the cells is considered to be a trigger for cancer.) Despite all of this, this organ is still an unbelievably patient customer. The liver does not react with pain even when it is ill, and it can still completely recover after severe damage. All of this leads us to underestimating its significance.

Practically every cancer patient shows a disturbed liver function and the pancreas and intestine are often also in a deplorable condition. People who drink alcohol, eat foods that are sweet, fat, and abundant, get little exercise, and also swallow medications are creating the greatest possible concerns for their liver. Like a hopelessly overburdened worker, it courageously tries to see it through. Its cries for help, such as weakness and a general sense of unwellness, remain unheard. Emotional crises (such as depression or burn-out) can develop and the entire body is endangered. Systemic diseases like cancer especially like to thrive on this fertile ground.

An unnatural lifestyle always primarily burdens the liver and then it can no longer adequately carry out its task as the guardian of biological equilibrium. We are therefore well advised to not simply overhear what our "silent" organ is telling us because liver care is the ultimate health care.

In a certain respect, **Padma Basic** also acts to protect the liver, which indirectly benefits cancer patients (see page 83).

THE CANCER OF THE SOUL

Someone once said: "Cancer is the laughter that was never laughed and the tears that were never cried."

Can a distressed soul cause cancer?

Although Western oncologists indignantly reject the concept of a "cancer personality," practitioners have without difficulty observed that, for example, depressive women much more frequently are afflicted by breast cancer than others. Many cancer patients without any significant risk factors demonstrate a tendency to suppress deeper feelings and emotional injuries. Yet, they continue to maintain the external intact world facade at any price. This is often accompanied by insufficient self-trust or the lack of supportive social relationships. It appears that the body is sending a signal here with "its" cancer, a cry for help. Tumors sometimes go into spontaneous remission as soon as a patient experiences more love and genuine attention. Be that as it may: Sensible "emotional hygiene" is a precondition for avoiding many illnesses, which certainly also includes cancer.

It may sound surprising, but a "strong" immune system continuously reports to the soul about its well-being and the reverse is just as true. We are whole, and everything is connected with everything else. This is exactly how the Tibetan medicine sees it. Its well-considered plant-medicine composition has an equally positive influence on both the body and the soul.

THE BATTLE ON SEVERAL FRONTS

As much as we may have discovered about the prevention and development of cancer: There is generally a large gap between knowledge and action in the practice. It is obvious that considerably more is invested in the "elimination" of cancer than in effective prevention models.

In the therapeutic area, there are currently a great many different approaches being tested. For example, there is an attempt to effect cancer tumors with the methods of gene technology using approaches like finding and blocking the genes that control growth. Or light-active substances are sent into the tumor in order to "heat" it and melt it by using laser rays. The most promising possibility seems to be interrupting the blood supply of cancerous tissue by taking away the support it receives from the neighboring cells. This is intended to occur through medications that switch off the specific cell signals and practically let the cancer "starve." Despite all of the enthusiasm, we should not overlook that fact that the above-mentioned methods always can only have an isolated effect on the cancer. In this process, the overall condition of the organism is usually not taken into consideration. Whether this is a wise approach is another matter.

Anyone who studies the possibilities offered by phytotherapy—especially some of the exotic plants—must realize that a potential of unimagined dimensions is slumbering here.

NATURAL REMEDIES AS AN OPPORTUNITY

Particularly in the industrial nations, it is becoming increasingly apparent that not only the aging process, but also our diets play an essential role in the development of cancer. Japanese immigrants in the USA provide a striking example of this. Their rate of breast and colon cancer increased dramatically as soon as they adopted the general American fast-food lifestyle. On the other hand, the religious group of the Mormons who lived in the Salt Lake City area, showed a very negligible rate of cancer rate in the American comparison. Their secret: They reject many of the "blessings" of civilization and nourish themselves as naturally as possible—without alcohol, tobacco, and other stimulants, eating very little meat and fat. They fast on a regular basis and exercise their bodies.[24]

THE HEALING FACTOR OF FOOD

The abundance that natural, health-bringing substances in our plant food has available can be seen in the table on pages 38-39. Many secondary phyto-chemicals have an effect as a cancer prophylaxis and provide immune stimulation. This should remind us of the **biophotons**, which move information from cell to cell at the speed of light. Biophysicists have discovered that the light content and the color spectrum of our food is just as important for health as the vitamins and other biosubstances. This coherent light radiation is greatest in fresh plant food, but very minimal in industrially processed foods. When we eat more "light," this contributes to the promotion of cell organization and to a continuous defiance of cancer. Cancer patients should not use instant meals, white sugar, and refined flour. These types of foods cannot satisfy the **"light-hunger"** of the cells and also impair the healthy intestinal activity. The same thing probably applies to the popular, convenient microwave meals.

So this approach eliminates the question regarding a "cancer diet." Such a diet does not exist because the consumption of high-quality plant foods is the decisive factor.

PADMA BASIC HELPS PREVENT METASTASES

The initial studies on the mechanism of action by Padma Basic in terms of cancer diseases took place at the *Hadassah University Hospital* in the vicinity of Jerusalem. The influence of this Tibetan herbal formula was tested relevant to breast cancer with the danger of metastases formation. The oncologist Professor Dr. Israel Vlodavsky was able to discover how Padma Basic contributes to stopping the formation of metastases through disseminated cancer cells.

As mentioned above, one isolated cancer tumor does not represent a deadly threat because it can be removed by an operation or even be kept in check with natural remedies. The dangerous factor is the daughter cells carried off by the blood stream. If these are not recognized and destroyed by the immune system, they will attach themselves to the inner wall of the blood vessels and attempt to break through them in order to reach the other organs. The tumor cells produce a special enzyme of their own for their purpose. Padma Basic apparently inhibits the formation of this special enzyme and therefore prevents the tumor cells from breaking larger pieces out of the walls of the vessels and decomposing them. The cancer cells are then forced to remain in the blood stream, where they are recognized and destroyed by the body's defense system. Since Padma Basic comprehensively strengthens the immune system at the same time, this offers an effective opportunity to meaningfully counteracting the spread of the cancer.[25]

MACROPHAGES—THE GARBAGE POLICE

B and T lymphocytes act as the cancer-fighters on the front lines. They directly attack the cancer tumor. On the other hand, the task of the phagocytes (macrophages and granulocytes) consists of "waste elimination." They practically eat everything that appears suspicious and exogenous to them. Experiments have revealed that macrophages are primarily responsible for the destruction of cancerous daughter cells. If there are many phagocytes found in the blood, metastases also occur less frequently. Because of the antioxidants it contains, Padma Basic not only functions as a radical-catcher, but also promotes the breakdown of molecules damaged by oxidation. Padma

Basic has been shown to strengthen the bio-radiation of the phagocytes and stimulate numerous chemical processes that facilitate their work.

The advantages of taking Padma Basic for cancer patients undergoing conventional medical therapies, as well as people with a high risk of disease are obvious in light of the above information. Additional studies with breast-cancer patients will soon be done in the USA (University of California). In addition, research will be done on the extent that Padma Basic can influence the growth of primary tumors. Since the development of a cancer tumor occurs in a way that is very similar to the growth of smooth muscle cells in arteriosclerosis, it would also be quite conceivable that Padma Basic has an additional inhibitory effect on the proliferation of primary cancer cells.

Padma Basic exerts a powerful anti-inflammatory effect and helps in the promotion of proper circulation. This can be very important in prevention of side-effects from radiation therapy, especially post-radiation fibrosis.

TIBETAN MEDICINES—
ALSO GOOD FOR THE SOUL?

There is a situation with which many of us are quite familiar: When we must bear a severe loss, when distress, worries, or aggravation weigh us down, then our physical health also suffers.

Suddenly, we are no longer as resistant against colds, we are plagued by backaches, have headaches, or feel tired all of the time.

This raises the question: Is our immune system weakened by sadness and other psychological stress (distress) weakened, possibly even "misprogrammed"? And, on the other hand, can contentment, balance, and joyful feelings (eustress) have a positive effect on our powers of resistance?

LATEST RESEARCH

About 20 years ago, there was an awakening of scientific interest in the complex correlations between the psyche, the hormonal balance, the immune and nervous system. This began in the USA and initiated a new area of research, **psycho-neuro-immunology (PNI).** It shows us perspectives that could decisively change the orientation of modern medicine in the future. Above all, the AIDS problem makes it clear that the care of the immune systems should be paramount in importance.

At the *University of Miami*, Dr. Michael Antoni compared the metabolic reactions of healthy and HIV-positive test subjects with the following result: The defense system of an AIDS-infected person reacts differently to stress than that of a healthy human being. However, the researchers not only looked at the antibodies and the immune reactions, but also wanted to more precisely illuminate the role of the soul. They had no doubts that it must be more than just an observer in the exciting game of life.

In his experiments, Dr. Antoni was able to determine that men who fell into a state of depression after the AIDS diagnosis lost the T helper cells much more quickly than the afflicted who reacted to their destiny with confidence and an active life. A high number of T helper cells can, as we now know, prevent the outbreak of the AIDS infection.[26]

However, the most astounding finding of all of the immunological studies was that our defense system does not, as had long been assumed, work "autonomously," meaning independently. Instead, its activities are closely linked with all of the other biochemical processes in the body. Dr. Robert Ader of the University of Rochester in New York discovered evidence in his laboratory experiments that our immune system is influenced by brain activity. However, this finding is already more than 2000 years old. The Greek physician Heraclitus had already claimed that our feelings control our health.[27]

MESSENGER SUBSTANCES AND PEPTIDES

The discovery of **neurotransmitters**, which are the substances that function as information-carriers between the brain and the nerve cells, has made the idea of the healing or destructive power of emotions socially acceptable. We now know for certain that the "biochemical alphabet" of the neurotransmitters is understood by all (!) of the body cells. Both thymus gland and the bone marrow and lymphatic tissue are permeated with fine nerve fibers whose "antennas" respond to any brain activity.

An advocate of this theory, Dr. David Felten of Rochester, supplied the first microscopic images of this biological wonder[28] and immediately attracted the ridicule of the professional world. How could it be possible that nerves "talked" with mobile cells? But precisely this situation is the case.

Our immune cells have, exactly like each individual nerve cell, the respective receptors for chemical messenger substances. This means that they can communicate with every part of the body, but especially with the brain. All of the messenger substances, no matter what their origin may be, have the same chemical structure. These are **peptides** (from the Greek word *eupeptos* = digestible). Peptides consist of short-chained amino acid and are produced not only in the brain and other organs, but also by the nervous, hormonal, or immune system and used as sources of information. In these neuropeptides, we can see the biochemical correlate of our feelings. They appear to be the bridge—the missing link, so to speak—between the body and the soul.

When Tibetan physicians now claim that their treatment procedures and medicines can benefit human beings in their physical-mental unity, they are solely imparting insights that are thousands of years old, which we now can finally prove in the scientific sense as well.

THE DIALOG OF LIFE

In order for our immune system to find the middle path between too little and too much stimulation, it requires various types of information that we supply to it not only from the outside world through our diet and environmental stimuli but also through our respective sensations.

Our defense cells respond promptly through their own **"immunotransmitters"** and inform the brain in turn of their own condition.

This cellular dialog can result in a disease-causing or healing effect, and it is largely up to us in terms of the content of the messages that are exchanged here. The expression "positive thinking" has increasingly degenerated into a mechanistic phrase. It indicates no specific techniques but means that it is enough for us to feel good and have a sense of security—that we simply don't let ourselves become discouraged. Then our immune system will also react with "purring."

WHEN THE SOUL COMMUNICATES WITH THE BODY

Many decades ago, an interesting test took place in the USA. The behavior and personal history of a number of trained physicians was examined. This showed that test subjects who tended toward depression and worries were much more frequently and more severely ill than those who had a well-adjusted "balance sheet of the soul."

Dr. Kathleen Dillon of Western New England College in Massachusetts also investigated the effect of feelings on the immune system. In her study, she showed students one funny film and one sad film. Afterward, the IgA levels in the saliva of the test subjects were determined. (High IgA levels mean greater powers of resistance against infections.) The results spoke for themselves. The hearty laughter of the young people in response to the funny film caused their IgA levels to increase dramatically, but the sad film had the opposite effect. In addition, it showed that the high IgA values were maintained the longest for the students who otherwise had a very healthy sense of humor.[29]

Similar results have been found in many other studies: Feelings of sadness and despair activate specific regions of the brain and also stimulate the adrenal glands at the same time. An increased amount of the stress-producing hormones are released. This keeps the immune system in a constant state of alert, until it is ultimately becomes exhausted. Feelings like hatred, anger, or aggravation trigger analogous physical reactions. On the other hand, joy, confidence, and love contribute to physical relaxation.

But the "physical approach" also works. Naturopathic therapies, relaxation gymnastics, and a healthy diet not only continuously improve the state of the immune system, but also the emotional state of a human being. In short: It is possible to therapeutically approach a health disorder, which always affects the entire patient, on various levels and prevent its consequences. In this sense, the care of the immune system is just as important as the (re)establishment of the emotional equilibrium. The psyche and soma—soul and body—mutually influence each other.

PADMA BASIC—ALSO GOOD FOR THE SOUL?

What works in one direction should also function the other way around. If the immune cells can understand the message of our feelings, why shouldn't it be possible to improve the emotional well-being by providing the body's defense system with strengthening impulses through a multi-substance mixture made of plants?

In the practice study involving 15 Swiss physicians and 147 patients that was evaluated in 2002 (see pages 63ff.), the recorded finding also indicated a positive effect of Padma Basic on the psychological well-being of the examined patients.

On the one hand, we can assume that patients with severe circulation disorders also experience an improvement in their emotional condition when their complaints subsided. On the other hand, the participants in the study clearly expressed that existing sleep disorders, anxiety, and depressive episodes slowly changed from intense to weak or stopped completely as a result of taking Padma Basic.

The observed relief of **tinnitus** (ringing in the ears) could, apart from the circulatory-supporting effects, also be a result of the comprehensive calming of the entire organism. This very oppressive "noise stress in the ear" may also frequently be related to excess emotional-mental pressure. Padma Basic can help in reducing this pressure. Furthermore, it is interesting that Chinese medicine also uses the acupuncture point *Mingmen*, which can also be used in conjunction with Padma Basic, for relieving ringing in the ears (for details, also see page 34).

PERSONAL EXPERIENCES WITH PADMA BASIC

Although personal opinion is considered subjective in scientific terms and therefore not applicable, I would also like to include my own positive experiences with Padma Basic at this point. It has even made a decisive contribution to the fact that you are holding this book in your hands at all.

I will openly admit that I am a woman who at times has had problems with nervousness. Now that I am more aware of the deeper causes, I can deal with things in a more relaxed manner. Taking Padma Basic as a food supplement on a regular basis has also greatly improved both my physical **and** emotional well-being. I am less frequently ill and feel more balanced and fit on the whole. This is my personal experience. You are completely at liberty, dear reader, to prove the truth of this statement for yourself at any time.

Padma Basic functions as a "cooling" formula to counter an "overheated" lifestyle with stress and the continual pressure to perform at high levels. This lifestyle very much requires a form of gentle regulation to compensate for the constant stimulation through external impulses. For these reasons, it is suitable as both a basic therapy for chronic fatigue syndrome (CFS), as well as for the often cited "burnout." According to reports, Padma Basic has already been called a very effective "stress pill for managers."

ADDITIONAL AREAS OF USE FOR PADMA BASIC

In the systematic indication list of the 14 Tibetan medicine specialties that Karl Lutz initially compiled together with the Study Group for Tibetan Medicine in Zurich the formula No. 28 (Padma Basic) occupies an outstanding position. Numerous application possibilities have been listed, and it is obvious that Padma Basic is being administered by physicians for many types of ailments in combination with other multi-substance mixtures from the list. Its use is always appropriate when there are acute or chronic infection or purulent infections. The formula No. 28 has been described as antibacterial, disinfectant, stimulating for the heart and circulation, and generally supportive of healing. It promotes the "purifying and nourishing property of the blood" and strengthens the "production of energy from the core" (Chinese description of how we absorb and utilize physical and mental food). As a result, this remedy is frequently used as a basic medication.[30]

In addition to the studies that have already been mentioned above, there are also individual research reports on Padma Basic in following areas:

USE IN CHRONIC-INFECTIOUS HEPATITIS B

Chronic hepatitis (inflammation of the liver) occurs as the result of an acute infection with the hepatitis virus that has not healed—and often has not even been recognized as such. There are two forms: a chronic-persistent (form) and the aggressive type. Both of these usually develop over a number of years and any treatment of them is protracted. In addition to localized pain, chronic hepatitis can severely impair the respective patient's functional capacity, even if the laboratory values are satisfactory.

Today we know that this chronic-inflammatory damage to the liver cells is based on a permanent immune reaction with viral antigens. The organism is in a constant state of alert, but it does not succeed in ultimately eliminating the infection of the hepatitis virus. In such cases, Padma Basic can bring relief and sometimes even healing, as shown by two studies from the years 1992 and 1993.

In a two-year test, 126 adults and 52 children with chronic hepatitis B received 3 times 2 tablets of Padma Basic every day. The result: In about 90% of the Test subjects, the immune regulation was measurably improved. In about 15%, there was no longer any cellular viral infection to be detected after this two-year period.

A second study with 34 test subjects resulted in similar positive results. In this study, two decisive advantages became apparent:

- Padma Basic improves the overall immune status, and
- The advancement of inflammatory processes is stopped.[31]

With Padma Basic, it is apparently possible to prevent lasting liver damage. The medical professional and author Dr. Egbert Asshauer has also reported on such a case: Because of a chronic infection with hepatitis B, a younger man suffered from constant fatigue and enlargement of the liver. Dr. Asshauer treated the patient with Padma Basic; seven months later, there was still an infection but no more evidence of liver damage.[32]

Dr. Asshauer also recommends the experimental application of Padma Basic in cases of chronic hepatitis C.[33]

A VOICE FROM POLAND

At the Washington congress in the year 1998, Professor Lech Hryniewicki from the Medical Academy of Poznan in Poland lectured on an open pilot study of 34 patients with active, chronic hepatitis B. After taking Padma Basic for several months, the virus antigen had completely disappeared in 18% of the patients and could not longer be detected in 33% of the virus DNS. 41% of the test subjects with an active liver cirrhosis discovered that it remained inactive after this treatment.

USE IN CHRONIC RESPIRATORY INFECTIONS AND ASTHMA

No mother will ever forget the time when her children came down with one cold after the other. From infancy to puberty, each runny nose is followed by the next cough. This "training" is usually good for the immune system and the healing occurs without complications, but many children can be observed to have a conspicuous weakness of the defense system.

There have primarily been two test series with Padma Basic that are interesting in this regard:

In tests with children of various age groups (younger than 3 years and up to 16 years) who are susceptible to infection and took Padma Basic for a time period of between six and ten weeks, the results were a distinct reduction in the number of chronic respiratory infections (for example, from recurrent bronchitis).

Children older than 3 years receive one tablet of Padma Basic 3 times a day; the younger ones received one-half of a table 3 times a day. In up to 70% of the cases, this therapy was effective.[34]

My own son can also serve as an example here: For years I have been giving him one tablet of Padma Basic twice daily during the time period from September until spring. The cold and cough periods, which used to last many weeks, are now part of the past. For more information on this topic, also see *Padma Flu Formula* and *Padma Cough Formula* (see page 100).

Padma Basic is, as the practice has shown, just as helpful against **chronic inflammations of the maxillary sinuses**—and especially when antibiotics no longer have an effect. It influences purulent processes and allows the inflammatory symptoms disappear.

There have not yet been adequate empiric findings established regarding the beneficial effect of Padma Basic in cases of **bronchial asthma**. However, since it has been shown that asthmatics have inflammatory cells in the lung area, it would certainly be worthwhile to test the use of Padma Basic (as a complementary therapy).

Padma Basic may also offer the same relief for **hay fever** and related allergic disorders of the immune system by inhibiting excessive reaction. Also see *Padma Sarsaparilla Formula* (page 102) for more information on this topic.

ADDITIONAL AREAS OF USE

Because of the effects discovered in experiments, in which the various diseases play a role, Padma Basic may also have a supportive effect in following cases (always solely as a supplementary, prescribed therapy and in consultation with the treating physician or health practitioner):

USE IN RHEUMATOID ARTHRITIS AND CHRONIC POLYARTHRITIS (INFLAMMATION OF THE JOINTS)

Above all, a study carried out by the University of Massachusetts on site in Dharamsala is remarkable in its examination of the effectiveness of conventional ant rheumatic agents in comparison to Tibetan medicine. The findings showed that the modern Western medications are—logically enough—superior when it comes to the alleviation of pain; however, the measures of Tibetan medicine (diet, plant medicines, etc.) were much more successful in restoring the functionality of the joints.[35] For more information on this, also see the new *Padma Rheumatism Acute Formula* (page 101).

Comparative studies such as this are especially emphatic in showing how much benefit comes from a combined application of old and new medical procedures in helping patients.

For more information about the so-called autoimmune disorders, see the chapter on "Padma Basic—The Motor of the Immune Systems".

OTHER AREAS OF USE

Padma Basic is also advisable for supportive treatment of local-inflammatory processes, including:

- Cystitis (urinary-tract inflammation)
- Gastroenteritis (inflammation of the gastrointestinal tract)
- Gingivitis (inflammation of the gums)
- Ulcus ventriculi and duodeni (gastric and duodenal ulcers)
- Ulcus cruris (open leg) and phlebitis (surface inflammation of a vein)

When there is a tendency toward furunculosis and the formation of abscesses in the healing phase of infectious diseases (including genuine influenza), as well as in accelerating the healing of wounds, specifically after operations.

There have also been reports of relieving **migraine** (especially those caused by hormones) with liver participation. (Incidentally, migraines are very successfully relieved by Tibetan physicians with jewel pills.)

Moreover, another study involved the experimental use of Padma Basic for cases of **multiple sclerosis.** In 44% of the patient group treated with Padma Basic, a distinct improvement of their general condition was observed (muscle power, remission of the sphincter disorders).[36]

In any of these cases, a physician/naturopath should be consulted, especially when a person must take some type of medication on a regular basis.

PADMA BASIC IN SPORTS

Top athletic performance and physical strain leave traces in the body that are comparable to an inflammatory state of exhaustion. This can lead to signs of wear and muscle and joint complaints. However, if the body is supplied with regulating impulses afterwards, such as that of the mixture of the medicinal herbs in Padma Basic, negative consequences can be avoided.

Because of its anti-inflammatory and circulation-supporting properties, Padma Basic is increasingly being used by athletes. Competitive athletes (such as marathon runners) report a decreased tendency toward inflammation of the mucous bursa and Achilles tendon. Fewer cramps and less muscle hardening occurs. The recovery after a competitive event takes place more quickly and without complications.

The physicians of the *Muttenz Sports Clinic* (Switzerland) have used Padma Basic for years and also apply it in postoperative care following orthopedic surgery. The remedy, according to Dr. Urs Martin, contributes toward the more rapid removal of inflammatory substances, which brings about a quicker healing of injuries.

Two Moroccan top ultra-marathon runners, the Ahansal brothers (multiple winners of the *Marathon des Sables*, which covers more than 145 miles in 6 days, and the Swiss Alpine Marathon) have been using Padma Basic for years. These top athletes report a shorter regeneration time, less cramping in the legs, and fewer inflammations. Lahcen Ahansal says: "Padma Basic is good for our regeneration. If we participate in many runs, we are in form again more quickly afterward. In our desert medicine we take herbs, too. With Padma Basic, these are conveniently packed in pills and that is great for us."

In this situation, Padma Basic has the effect of a natural and gentle restorative agent that optimally supports the organism in its regeneration phase after athletic activities.

Padma Basic is naturally not a remedy for directly increasing performance; instead, it is a gentle "legal doping" for the immune system. As a result, all of the body functions are harmonized and the powers of self-healing are stimulated.

The recommended dosage is between 2 and 6 tablets per day, depending upon the training intensity.

PADMA LAX

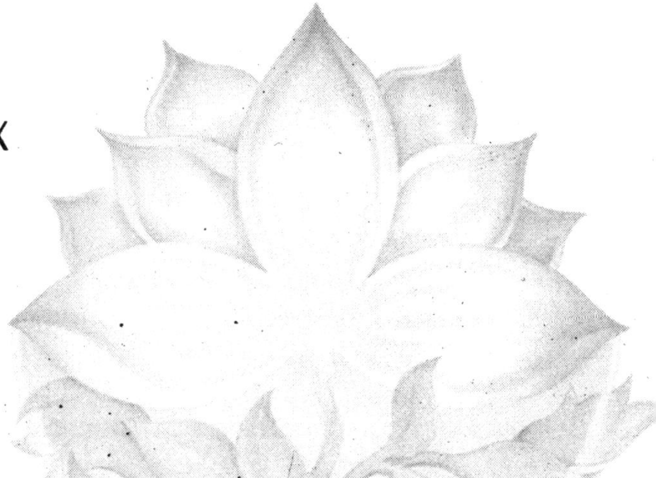

Because of the very triumphant advance that Padma Basic has started as the "basic therapeutic preparation" of the Tibetan plant medicine, the other Tibetan medicine in standardized form on the market (also available in the US) is often overlooked. Padma Lax is traditionally indicated as a mild, well-tolerated laxative (medicinal remedy with purgative effect)—which its name already indicates.

HELP FOR SLUGGISH INTESTINES

"Death lives in the intestine": This is a radical statement, but it is literally true.

As long as all of the eliminatory functions of our body work without a complaint, we stay healthy and feel full of life. Unfortunately, going to the toilet on a regular basis is wishful thinking for a great number of people. Most of the afflicted individuals refuse to believe how much the modern, hectic lifestyle and common improper nutrition contribute to this problem. The use of chemical laxatives is increasing and many people have completely lost a sense of the natural eliminatory processes. Instead of a pleasant cleansing of the body, they are only seen as a necessary evil that disturbs the over-scheduled course of our day. No wonder that things stop "moving smoothly" at some point.

NOT A PETTY OFFENSE

Occasional or severe constipation (obstipation) is the most widespread calamity of modern civilization. However, when we realize that the inner walls of the intestines would cover a surface of about 200 (!) square meters if they were spread out, the problem becomes quite clear: Neglect cannot remain without consequences in this area.

If the contents of the intestines are not eliminated on a regular basis, harmful substances can return to the blood and lymphatic circulation—after all, the intestinal walls are permeable—and flood the entire body with cellular toxins from there. This is also why "continuously constipated" patients usually also have a poor skin appearance, suffer from diffuse headaches, and just simply do not feel good on the whole.

This makes it clear: Constipation is not a harmless "petty offense."

But the causes for it are usually quite obvious. In order to help the intestine do its daily work, an emphasis should be placed upon the following measures: adequate roughage, which is contained in fruit, vegetables, and whole-grain products (an additional, completely harmless aid for better digestion is psyllium husks, which can be purchased in natural food stores and health food stores). The abundant intake of fluids through spring water, tea (herb teas, green tea, Rooibos tea, etc.), diluted fruit or vegetable juices, and soup is important. Some cases of constipation can be cured through these measures alone.

In addition, it is necessary to engage in a minimum amount of exercise and avoid excessive stress. It is also important for individuals to learn to say no—and mean it—when they are overworked. The impulse to defecate should never be ignored, for example, by children who do not want to interrupt a game. Incidentally, according to the biological clock the best "emptying times" are between 5 a.m. and

7 a.m. or 5 p.m. and 7 p.m. During these phases of the day, the body is prepared for maximum cleansing.

THE BRAIN IN THE BELLY

If anyone ever accuses you of "acting from the gut" take it as a compliment since this is the right way to do things. As already mentioned in the chapter on Padma Basic and the soul, nothing occurs in an isolated way in the body. Our intestine processes not only food, it must also deal with the emotional burdens. Its nerve tissue is so sensitive that we can actually consider this area to be the body's "**second brain.**" There is definitely a reason why we have such expressions as "this problem is giving me a bellyache" or "that is hard for me to digest."

A tense intestine becomes hardened and cramped; it halts its peristalsis (natural wave movement) and no longer wants to "let go" of anything. In this situation, the digestion can be helped out with plant remedies, but it is also important to simultaneously look for a solution to possibly emotional tensions.

PADMA LAX HAS A GENTLE AND SURE EFFECT

Based on the fundamentals of Tibetan medicine described at the beginning, Padma Lax is also a combination of 15 plant and mineral components that, despite the low dosage, ensure an optimal effectiveness. The main components help the intestine to once again become active, while the other ingredients generally support the digestive process, induce the expulsion of gas (carminative), relieve cramps (antispasmodic), and protect the mucous membrane.

From the Tibetan perspective, Padma Lax promotes the "digestive heat." It brings the three body energies back into harmony since only an intact "digestive fire" guarantees well-being and vitality.

IMPORTANT APPLICATION INFORMATION·

Padma Lax is suitable for the short-term treatment of constipation without any special diagnosis. It should not be used if there is stomach pain of an unclear origin, a suspicious of intestinal obstruction, irritation of the appendix.

Pregnant and breastfeeding women and children under twelve years of age should not take Padma Lax. Like any type of laxative, Padma Lax could possibly trigger contractions. Specific substances that it contains (antrachinons) find their way into the breast milk, and the possible consequences of this for the baby have not been clarified. In these cases, it is better to use the harmless psyllium seeds in connection with the Padma tea "After Meal" (for more details, see the chapter on "Tibetan Teas—A Simple Way to Achieve Well-Being").

The normal dosage is one tablet with abundant fluids (water, tea) taken before bedtime. The effect will then become evident after about eight hours, in the morning. In stubborn cases, two tablets per day are appropriate, but the dosage should be reduced as soon as possible. In no case is Padma Lax intended to be used continually in full dosage or as an aid in losing weight. The result of such misuse could be a dangerous loss of fluids and mineral substances. Once you regain normal and regular bowl movements, the maintenance dosage for Padma Lax can be reduced to 2-3 tablets per week. In about 1/3 of subjects, bowl movements will remain regular without any need to use Padma Lax.

In addition, caution is required when simultaneously taking heart remedies, diuretic medications, and corticoadrenal hormones (corticosteroids). Especially when used over a longer period of time, Padma Lax could strengthen or change their effects. Always consult a physical in these cases!

If a mild diarrhea should occur while taking Padma Lax, reduce the dosage and drink plenty of liquids. On the other hand, occasional red coloration of the urine is normal and no cause for concern.

HOPE FOR THE IRRITABLE COLON SYNDROME

This disorder has many names: irritable colon (Colon irritabile), irritable bowel syndrome (IBS), spastic colon, or colitis mucosa. Approximately 20% of the Western population suffers from this. Women are more frequently affected than men (perhaps because they live more "from their guts"). Organic causes are not detectable in the irritable colon syndrome. In addition to possible allergies to specific foods, primarily emotional causes are presumed to trigger it. Among the symptoms are abdominal cramps and flatulence, heartburn, frequent alternating between diarrhea and constipation, as well as backache, circulatory weakness and "nervous" palpitation (heart consciousness). An irritated digestive tract involves the entire body. The relevance of the irritable-colon problem is shown by the fact that this diagnosis constitutes 50% of all digestive disorders causing patients to seek help. Many cannot even work because of the pain, which is almost unbearable. In addition to the above-mentioned measures for taking care of the intestines, Padma Lax also appears to be beneficial in these cases.

Recently, a placebo-controlled double-blind study on the topic of constipation-caused irritable colon was carried out by Dr. Sarah Sallon and her team at the *Hadassah University Hospital* in Jerusalem (see also pages 74f.). Padma Lax was tested for the treatment of patients with a constipation-caused IBS. 80 patients with this disease were randomized and treated either with Padma Lax or a placebo. Those using Padma Lax showed a remarkable improvement of the symptoms. 70% of the patients who had taken the Padma Lax experienced a general improvement of the intestinal activity (as opposed to 11% in the untreated placebo group). 76% stated that they distinctly preferred this therapy to the previous treatment attempts. They had experienced a clear decrease in the severe abdominal pain and flatulence.

It is interesting that Padma Lax is apparently not habit-forming, as is the case for many laxatives, especially plant-based remedies. The side-effects (10 of 34 patients) were quite minor. They were expressed in a slight increase in the occurrence of diarrhea; however, this disappeared after a reduction of the dosage. Moreover, the use of Padma Lax did not cause any intensive, radical elimination of the intestines, which is usually connected with a dangerously high loss of water and mineral substances. In addition to a more gentle elimination, this remedy also stimulates digestion and helps the body find its way back to normal functioning.[37]

For individuals whose intestine constantly reacts in an "irritable" manner, it is high time to get help in the form of these natural vital substances. Padma Lax provides "first aid" in such cases. Once things have improved after one to two weeks, the digestive system can be given additional meaningful support with the Tibetan tea mixtures *"After Meal"* and *"At Any Time"* or through the new *"Padma Digestive Tonic"* (for more information see pages 101 and 115ff.).

Contents of Padma Lax

Scientific Name	Common Name	Content in Milligram (mg) per Tablet
Zingiber officinale	Ginger rhizome	70.00
Rheum palmatum	Chinese rhubarb root	70.00
Rhamnus frangula	Frangula bark	52.50
Rhamnus purshiana	Cascara sagrada bark	52.50
Gentiana lutea	Gentian root	35.00
Terminalia chebula	Chebulic myrobalan	35.00
Inula helenium	Elecampane root	35.00
Sodium sulfate	Sodium sulfate	35.00
Kaolin	Heavy kaolin	25.00
Sodium bicarbonate	Sodium bicarbonate	15.00
Aloe vera and/or Aloe ferox	Aloe extract	12.50
Jateorhiza palmata	Calumba root	10.00
Marsdenia cundurango	Condurango bark	10.00
Piper longum	Long pepper	3.50
Strychnos nux-vomica	Nux-vomica seed	1.75

Source: EcoNugenics, Inc. (see page 149)

NEW HEALING REMEDIES FROM THE TRADITION OF TIBETAN MEDICINE

From the years 2001 to 2003, *Padma* introduced to the market a total of 14 additional remedies, based on ancient original Tibetan formulas—initially in the Swiss Canton of Appenzell Ausserrhoden.

IN PROVEN QUALITY

Like all Tibetan medicines, the new Padma formulas consist of natural, high-quality raw substances. Because of their well-conceived composition, they are suitable for restoring the equilibrium of the "three subtle energies" (Wind, Bile, and Phlegm) in the body when there are various complaints.

The careful composition of the main and the secondary components optimizes the desired therapeutic effect. These raw materials come exclusively from plants and minerals that have been subjected to strict quality inspections before they are carefully compressed into the time-tested tablet form. There are also no dyes, preservatives, or taste-correcting substances in the "new Padmas." As we know, the smell and taste are an essential factor for the effect of the Tibetan remedies.

FROM LACK OF APPETITE TO CRAMPS IN THE CALVES OF THE LEGS

For a great variety of health disorders, the new *Padma* formulas represent a suitable form of immediate aid that can be ideally supplemented in the healing stage by Padma Basic as an immune-stimulator.

Padma Flu Formula: Developed from the original *Kyung nga* formula. Has a balancing and healing effect in the acute stages and during the short-term follow-up treatment of flu and influenza infections. It provides support for the body in the control of pathogens. Do not use for children under 12 years of age.

Padma Cough Formula: Original *rGun 'brum 7* (pronounced: *Gundum dunba**) formula.

Loosens sticky phlegm and has a mildly warmly effect on the respiratory passages in cases of (hacking) cough and bronchitis. Also suitable for children.

Padma Heartburn Formula: Original *Cong zhi 6* (pronounced: *Chong zhi dugba**) formula.

Helps in cases of heartburn and acid reflux; the sharp taste is an indispensable active component. For children under 12 years of age, use only after consulting a medical professional.

Padma Bowel Regulator: Original *Zhi byed 6* (pronounced: *Zhi je dugba**) formula.

Effective against digestive disorders (diarrhea/constipation) caused by too little "inner heat"; against a sensation of fullness, pressure over the stomach, and after eating questionable foods. Do not use during pregnancy and the lactation period.

* pronounced "u" as in "put"

Padma Digestive Tonic: Original *Se 'bru 5* (pronounced: *Sedu ngaba**) formula.

Helps maintain normal digestive fire, relieves flatulence and a feeling of fullness after meals. This is also suitable as a preventative remedy, as well as relieving cold hands and feet caused by "stomach coldness".

Padma Rheumatism Acute Formula: Original *Le tre 5* (pronounced: *Le tre ngaba*) formula.

Anti-inflammatory in cases of acute rheumatic complaints, joint swelling, and muscle pain; also relieves gout and arthritis. It is also definitely recommended to try it for the increasingly frequent symptoms of fibromyalgia (generalized tendomyopathy—"everything-hurts syndrome"). For children under 12 years of age, use only after consulting a medical professional. Do not take longer than 2 months without an interruption.

Padma Liver-Gallbladder Tonic: Comes from the group of the *Garnag* formulas.

Helpful against functional weakness of the liver and gallbladder with symptoms such as fatigue, lack of appetite, nausea, as well as migraines related to the liver. For the follow-up treatment of liver inflammations. For children under 12 years of age, use only after consulting a medical professional.

Padma Liver Regulator: Original *'Bras bu 3 thang* (pronounced: *De bu sum thang**) formula.

Cools and harmonizes the "three energies," mildly stimulates the intestinal activity. Symptoms as for *Padma Liver-Gallbladder Tonic*, especially for the follow-up treatment of liver inflammation and insufficient liver function.

Padma Urinary-Tract Formula: Belongs to the group of the classic *A ru* (pronounced: *A ru**) formulas.

Has a diuretic and disinfecting effect; relieves acute, uncomplicated urinary-tract infections. Also suitable for the prevention of bladder inflammations and bladder irritations. If fever occurs, always consult a physician! This remedy corresponds to the Tibetan medicine *Urotib* (see pages 105ff.).

Padma Vein Tonic: Developed in cooperation with Tibetan physicians for the support of water elimination and tonifying the vein walls in cases of varicose veins, small varicose dilatations of the cutaneous veins, swollen legs, pain, and a feeling of heaviness. Also helpful against cramps of the calves and hemorrhoids. Not suitable for children under 12 years of age.

Padma Sarsaparilla Formula: Belongs to the group of the *Tufuling* (pronounced: *Toofooling*) formulas.

Against allergies and for detoxification, made according to the instructions of the Buryat Tibetan physician Dr. Dougar ov.

Padma Cold Formula: Original *Nor bu 7 thang* (pronounced: *Norbu du tang**) formula.

This classical formula is used for coughs and sneezes, flu with symptoms like fever, colds, sinusitis, sore throat, muscle pain, as well as for the burn-out syndrome.

Padma Nerve Formula: Original *Srog 'zin 10* (pronounced: *Sogzin chuba**) formula. This classical formula has a relaxing and nervine effect on nervousness, tension, irritability, and restlessness.

Padma Menstrual Cycle Formula: Original *Zlatsen 'khrugs sel* (pronounced: *Dhatsen trugsel**) formula.

This formula has a warming and spasmolytic effect on the lower abdomen. It supports women during the premenstrual and menstrual phase of the cycle.

For additional information about availability in the USA and Canada contact EcoNugenis, Inc. For other countries, contact *Padma* (see page 149).

UROTIB—
HELP FOR A BURNING PROBLEM

Surveys in Western countries show that inflammations of the urogenital tract, which means the bladder and the urinary tract, are among the most frequent health problems. About one-half of all women have had these types of problems at some time in their lifetime, and every fifth woman has had them even more than once. However, this unpleasant and often protracted disease also afflicts men. It most frequently affects the older male generation.

Infections of the urogenital system find a fertile ground when foreign microorganisms are deposited in urethra or urinary bladder and cause burning pain during urination. This is usually accompanied by an intensified urge to urinate and, if the kidneys are also afflicted, backache as well.

At this point, it should be emphasized that a physician should immediately be consulted to clarify the diagnosis in the following cases. Get an expert's opinion when:

- There is blood in the urine
- Pain occurs in the back or lower abdomen that continues for days or continually returns
- The complaints are accompanied by nausea, vomiting, or fever.

FLUIDS ARE IMPORTANT

One rule for all of these types of infections, which is ignored much too often, is: Drink enough fluids! Sufficient drinking—and the best choice is good spring water—helps in quickly eliminating harmful germs. This healing process for inflammatory diseases of the urinary organs can be effectively supported by a plant multi-substance preparation. This appears to be even more important since the widespread application of antibiotics against urinary tract infections rarely promises lasting success. In 80% of the afflicted, the ailment stubbornly returns again.

AN ADDITIONAL MESSENGER OF THE GENTLE VARIETY

Although it is not a member of the "*Padma* family," the plant remedy *Dr. Andres Urotib* can also be classified as an original Tibetan medicine. Until recently, it was only on the market through the Swiss pharmacy in Zurich, but now it can also be obtained in other countries through pharmacies. *Urotib* corresponds with the *Padma Urinary Tract Formula* (see pages 101f.).

Like all Tibetan herbal remedies, *Urotib* is a complex mixture of active substances. Its positive effects are based on the synergy principle, which means that they occur through the perfect interplay of carefully coordinated plant components. The herbal tablets are naturally free of artificial dyes and preservatives or stabilizers

Urotib herbal tablets generally have a pain-relieving, urine-disinfecting, and diuretic effect. They are suited as a (supplementary) treatment of kidney and bladder inflammations, as well as similar disorders.

The indications include in particular:

- Urethritis (inflammation of the urethra)
- Pyelonephritis (inflammation of the kidney and its pelvis)
- Nephrosis (non-inflammatory, degenerative kidney disease)
- Nephrolithiasis (calculi in the kidneys)

When drinking the appropriate amounts of liquids, *Urotib* simultaneously promotes the elimination of urinary-tract sediments (gravel, small stones) in a natural way. However, in such cases, this should always be discussed with the treating physician!

RECOMMENDATIONS FOR TAKING UROTIB

At the beginning, take 2 to 3 times 2 tablets of *Urotib* every day before meals together with a large quantity of fluids (1 cup of water). After a few days, when the inflammatory complaints have subsided, reduce the amount taken to 1-2 tablets per day. This dosage should be maintained until the complaints are completely healed. When used according to directions, *Urotib* has no undesired side-effects.

Note: Pregnant or lactating women should be careful when taking any type of medicinal remedies. In these cases, always consult a trusted physician before doing so.

Urotib can also be given to children over six years of age. However, be sure to consult a physician beforehand.

FREQUENTLY ASKED QUESTIONS

In this chapter, you will find additional information and answers to questions that frequently arise in relation to the applications of Padma Basic and Padma Lax.

How do I take Padma Basic at the right dosage?

Start with 1 tablet twice daily for three days. Then increase to 2 tablets, twice daily for three days and finally increase to the recommended dosage of 2x3/day. For mild cases of arteriosclerosis, results can be obtained with a dosage of 2x2/day. Continue the therapeutic dosage for 2-4 months. Once you observe a noticeable improvement that remains stable for a few weeks, reduce your dosage to 2x2/day for 1-2 months and then to a maintenance dosage of 1x2/day. As a food supplement or maintenance dose, take 1 tablet 1-2 times daily on an ongoing basis. There are no known side-effects for long-term applications.

For existing complaints (for example, advanced arteriosclerosis) take 2 tablets, 3 times a day, preferably at least 30-45 minutes before meals.

According to the principles of Tibetan medicine, it is important to consciously smell and taste Padma Basic when taking it, which means that the tablets should first be chewed and then swallowed with plenty of fluids (1-2 glasses of lukewarm spring water, tea, or milk). However, most people find it too difficult. You will still get the results if you swallow the tablets with water. This is the method that was commonly tested in the various clinical trials. If you want to take Padma Basic after meals, then wait at least 2 hours after eating. Although taking it during meals was originally discouraged, this is better in individual cases than not taking it at all because of intolerability.

If you take Padma Basic along with other medications, it is advisable but not absolutely necessary to take it separately from other medications (up to 1-2 hours before or after).

What should I observe when taking Padma Lax?

You can find the exact instructions in the respective chapter.

How long should I take Padma Basic?

As you know by now, many Tibetan herbal medicines have a slower and milder effect than chemical medications. This is gentler on the organism and offers some advantages.

You will notice on your own exactly when an improvement occurs and which dose you require to maintain it. You should give it at least four months before deciding that it doesn't work for you. You may also notice that you suddenly don't want to take it anymore. This is also an indication from your body that you should not ignore. However, Padma Basic is an exceptional medication in that it supports the organism so gently that no disadvantages can be expected when taking it on a long-term basis.

Are there side-effects and/or interactions with other medications?

According to previous experiences, Padma Basic does not influence or change the effects of other medications or natural remedies. In the same way, it also does not cause undesired side-effects. If slight digestive disorders (such as belching) occur, this can normally be eliminated by drinking enough fluids. In this case, possibly taking the tablets with the main meals is recommended. Only in isolated cases, certain individuals could not take Padma Basic because of an insurmountable aversion. However, this may be because our pampered gustatory nerves simply reject everything to which we are not accustomed. In this case, we must decide what is more important to us.

If you must take other medications, be sure to discuss the application of Padma Basic in every case with your physician.

Once your well-being has noticeably improved—for example, in the case of arterial circulatory disorders—then the dosage of the prescribed medicine can be appropriately adjusted.

I am a diabetic. Am I allowed to take Padma Basic?

Yes. There are no known contra-indications. Studies have indicated that Padma Basic has a positive effect on the glucose levels.

What should be observed during pregnancy and the breastfeeding period?

According to the previous studies, there is no reason not to take Padma Basic during this time. Please observe the measures that have already been mentioned (adequate drinking, etc.) and, when in doubt, consult your physician. In general, it is recommended to minimize the ingestion of herbal products during pregnancy unless you are under the supervision of a trained health professional with clinical experience in treating pregnancy with herbs.

In terms of **Padma Lax**, please remember that women who are pregnant or breastfeeding should not use this formula for safety's sake.

Can Padma Basic also be given to children?

According to the medical information, Padma Basic can be given without concern even to small children. Incidentally, it is free of gluten and lactose (important in cases of celiac disease or an intolerance to milk). The dosage depends upon the age and/or weight of the child. Usually, 1 tablet a day is completely adequate as prophylaxis for bigger children; for complaints, give 1 tablet 2 to 3 times a day. For smaller children (four years and younger), one-half of a tablet each time should be enough. Let it disintegrate in one tablespoon of water and then mix it into a porridge. Bigger children are quite willing to chew the tablets, and they often have a very fine sense of what helps them. However, if your child is completely opposed to taking Padma Basic, you should take this seriously as well. What may be good for many people may still not be the right thing for everyone.

Is it worthwhile to follow specific dietary guidelines as long as I take Tibetan medicines?

Apart from the suggestions in the individual chapters of this book, the original document of the Study Group for Tibetan Medicine recommends avoiding the following foods as much as possible while taking Tibetan herbal remedies:

- Animal fats (fatty meat, lard, whole milk, too much butter)
- Refined sugar
- Eating milk products directly after a meal of meat.
- The consumption of iced soft drinks (sodas), raw fruit, and juices should also be limited—especially when the weather is cold because of their cooling value.

On the other hand, the following is recommended:

- Drinking good high-quality spring water (no ice!)

- The moderate consumption of sour milk products (plain yogurt, kefir, sour milk/curds)

These suggestions serve the better tolerance of Tibetan plant remedies in general. It would therefore certainly be advantageous to observe them.

Can I take Padma Basic in addition to other naturopathic remedies?

Since there are no known interactions with other remedies for Padma Basic, this should be possible. But please observe the following: In order to be able to properly evaluate the effect of a natural remedy, it should first be used on its own. Although there are no empiric findings on the simultaneous ingestion of high-quality natural food supplements (such as bee pollen, micro-algae, raw molasses, and the like), there should hardly be any harm in taking them at the same time.

In the documentary film *The Knowledge of Healing* (see page 119), an enthusiastic user from the Swiss mountains tells of how additionally taking garlic capsules presumably supported the effect of Padma Basic against arteriosclerosis in his case.

So you basically must determine what you tolerate and what is good for you on your own. You can naturally always drink the Tibetan teas as well.

Where can I obtain Padma Basic, Padma Lax and the new Padma formulas?

For additional information about the availability contact EcoNugenis, Inc. in the USA and Canada. In other countries, contact *Padma* (see page 149).

TIBETAN TEAS—
A SIMPLE WAY
TO ACHIEVE WELL-BEING

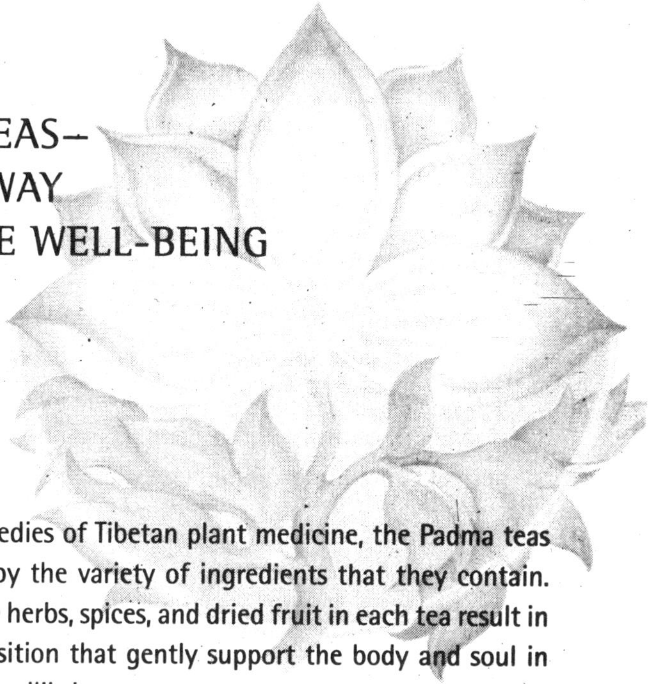

Like all of the remedies of Tibetan plant medicine, the Padma teas are distinguished by the variety of ingredients that they contain. Between 21 and 30 herbs, spices, and dried fruit in each tea result in a balanced composition that gently support the body and soul in finding a natural equilibrium.

Four special tea formulas have been composed by the manufacturing company in cooperation with **Dr. Kalsang Shak,** a Tibetan physician and tea expert who lives in Switzerland, according to the principles of the Tibetan teachings on health. Individual, ready-to-use tea bags guarantee that every cup of Padma tea has the same quality in an unchanging relationship of mixture ingredients.

PADMA TEA ANY TIME (DAILY TEA "DASHI-DELEK," ACCORDING TO DR. SHAK)

As the name already implies: This composition of 25 herbs, spices, and fruits has a balancing and harmonizing effect. In the hectic pace of everyday life, this tea can help us maintain our sense of inner peace and serenity. When enjoyed during the day, it helps ease the consequences of a general over-stimulation (the Tibetans speak of Wind disorders). As an evening tea, it promotes healthy sleep and calms the nerves. The "yellow" Padma tea is an ideal drink at work, but is just as suitable as the "house tea" for the entire family.

Ingredients:

Rose hips, raspberry leaves, sesame seeds, aniseed, stinging nettle, fennel, pomegranate seeds, ginger, chamomile flowers, cardamom, coriander, linden blossoms, peppermint, celery, licorice, cinnamon, caraway, cloves, cumin, jasmine blossoms, black pepper, saffron, nutmeg, long pepper, asafetida.

PADMA TEA AFTER MEAL (DIGESTION TEA "METOE," ACCORDING TO DR. SHAK)

The 24 harmoniously coordinated ingredients of this tea ideally support the process of the food absorption and utilization. Taken after meals, the components encourage pleasant relaxation and promote *Metoe*, the inner digestive fire. The "blue" Padma tea harmonizes Bile and Phlegm, helping balanced some of the disadvantages of our fast-paced modern age. Unfortunately, hastily eaten meals and an imbalanced diet are often part of our everyday lives. In these situations, the Padma tea *After Meal* can have a regulating effect. It works against "stomach-cold" (after too much raw foods or cold drinks) and helps in the digestion of unaccustomed foods (vacation!).

Ingredients:

Pomegranate seeds, lesser galangal, ginger, peppermint, black cumin, Szechwan pepper, fennel, wormwood, licorice, ajowan, dill seeds, aniseed, cardamom, caraway, cloves, cinnamon, coriander, bay leaves, chamomile flowers, fenugreek seeds, long pepper, black pepper, sodium bicarbonate (baking soda—acid regulator), nutmeg, asafetida.

PADMA TEA ON COLD DAYS (WINTER TEA "GOENKA," ACCORDING TO DR. SHAK)

Especially during the cold seasons, this tea mixture with 30 select components helps the body in maintaining its inner heat. The very pleasant-tasting "red" Padma tea can be used effectively for the prevention of colds and during the flu period. It strengthens the immune system and is an ideal winter drink. Moreover, it is also good to drink it whenever you suffer from inner "freezing," which may also be the case during time of extreme exhaustion or illness—independent of the season. It is also helpful for a weak constitution because of insufficient "digestive heat." From the Tibetan perspective, the Padma tea *On Cold Days* harmonizes the Phlegm energy.

Ingredients:

Apricot seeds, rose hips, ajowan, aniseed, safflowers, ginger, cumin, almonds, sesame seeds, sunflower seeds, licorice, lemon peel, fennel, Szechwan pepper, basil, fenugreek seeds, cloves, chamomile flowers, cardamom, coriander, turmeric, long pepper, linden blossoms, bay leaves, peppermint, Greek sage, black pepper, thyme, white mustard, cinnamon.

PADMA TEA FOR WOMEN (WOMEN'S TEA "DATSEN," ACCORDING TO DR. SHAK)

The composition of the Padma "lady's tea" takes into account the special needs of the female organism. Its 21 components gently support the natural regulatory mechanisms and help promote physical and emotional well-being.

The various complaints before and during menstruation can be distinctly eased by the Padma *For Women* tea. Especially the days before the period, the infamous premenstrual syndrome, are making life difficult for increasingly more women. The "orange" Padma tea can gently, but surely, help promote a consistent regulation in this case. This balanced drink is also a good remedy for the problems related to menopause (change of life) and may positively influence a wide range of related feelings of ill-health.

Incidentally, the symptom complex of the "change of life" is unknown to Tibetan medicine. Above all, this bundle of complaints is seen as a consequence of our Western, stress-oriented lifestyle.

Ingredients:

Cranberries, pomegranate seeds, caraway, fennel, raspberry leaves, ginger, turmeric, cloves, chamomile flowers, cardamom, coriander, cumin, peppermint, licorice, cinnamon, parsley, fenugreek seeds, nutmeg, asafetida, saffron.

Padma teas give us the possibility of experiencing the gentle but lasting effects of Tibetan medicine in an enjoyable way within the context of everyday life.

For additional information about the availability contact EcoNugenis, Inc. in the USA and Canada. In other countries, contact *Padma* (see page 149).

CASE HISTORIES–
THIS IS HOW PADMA BASIC HELPED ME

For more than eight years now, the German state-owned television station ARD has broadcast the afternoon talk show *Fliege* as an ambassador of gentle medical paths of healing. About once a week, the "Television Pastor" Juergen Fliege presents a great variety of naturopathic topics, allowing not only patients and healers but also renowned scientists and physicians to speak their minds. The very experienced physician and medical historian Professor Dr. Hans Schadewaldt has long been a regular on the show as a critical but very open representative of conventional medicine.

IT BEGAN ON THE "FLIEGE" SHOW

At the beginning of 1998, Tibetan medicine was the subject of a *Fliege* health program. The following guests appeared on the show: In addition to the film director Franz Reichle, the producer of the documentary film *The Knowledge of Healing* and the biophysicist Dr. Schwabl, there was also Mr. Wolfgang B. The doctors had given this patient, who suffered from severe coronary sclerosis (hardening of the arteries of the coronary vessel), three bypasses and then sent him into early retirement. Tibetan medicine became his salvation.

FROM THE HOSPITAL BED TO THE BICYCLE

Considering his circumstances, Mr. B could naturally no longer continue working as a plumber. Despite his recovery from the operations, his health condition was rapidly deteriorating. The heart bypasses that had been implanted became obstructed time and again. As a last possibility, he was offered the prospect of a very risky laser treatment or even heart transplantation. Mr. B. was in despair.

Then an acquaintance's daughter, who had seen the film *The Knowledge of Healing*, told him about Padma Basic. Although he was a declared proponent of conventional Western medicine, Mr. B. decided to try it. And, believe it or not: After about two months, his heart pain subsided and he was ultimately able to once again go on a two-hour walking tour. Today, as he says, Mr. B . walks "a mile or two almost every day to do his shopping" and rides up to 15 miles on his bike. His cardiologist could not believe the results and asked Mr. B. whether he had sent his twin brother instead. The physician had never heard of Padma Basic and did not consider it to be effective since "only Bayer and Hoechst have the right medications ..."

AND "FLIEGE" ONCE AGAIN

The same television show in which Mr. B. described his recovery also became a turning point for Mr. Hermann H. After three heart attacks, his condition was rapidly deteriorating despite good medical treatment that included a bypass operation. While watching *Fliege* he had heard of Padma Basic and obtained this Tibetan remedy for himself. After just a few weeks, he no longer needed the nitrogen spray and his blood levels were once again in the optimal range. This improvement was lasting.

The fact that Tibetan medicine is reaching a larger audience for the first time in Europe is due to a man who actually went to East Siberia because of an ecological project: the Swiss film director Franz Reichle. When he later researched Buddhism in a monastery, he came across the ancient Tibetan medicine there and it quickly became clear to him: "This is not hocus-pocus."

Although he first found the Swiss company *Padma, Inc.* while doing his subsequent research for the film *The Knowledge of Healing* back in his homeland, of all places, he had already experienced the astonishing effectiveness of Tibetan herbal pills on his own body.

RENAL COLIC AND DYSENTERY CURED

In 1994, Franz Reichle was in Moscow and developed severe kidney problems. However, instead of going to the American Clinic, he had himself treated by a Tibetan physician. Once he was back in Switzerland, the new x-rays showed no kidney damage of any type.

In the same year, Reichle contracted dysentery in India and was able to cure it with just one single Tibetan jewel pill. Within one day, this pill stopped the diarrhea and, one week later, all signs of the illness had been eliminated. Through the production of his documentary film, Franz Reichle learned not only to understand the gentle rhythms of the Buddhist way of life but he also knows today: "Everything has its own quality—also in medicine."

SAT 1 ALSO REPORTS

On March 18th, 2002 the TV physician Samuel Stutz treated the topic of Tibetan medicine in his program *1x Taeglich* (1x Daily). The guests in the studio were: Dr. Ruedi Andres of the Stadelhofen-Apotheke (pharmacy) of Zurich, as well as Ms. Rosmarie S., an arteriosclerosis patient. After some fundamental explanations by Dr. Andres on the herbal formula Padma Basic, Ms. S. told the story of her illness:

Because of a vascular occlusion on the right leg, she had been operated three times since 1997. Despite these operations, the arteriosclerosis was advancing without mercy and she was threatened with having her leg amputated. The right foot no longer showed a pulse; it was white and cold, and she could hardly walk any more.

On her own, the patient then began to take Padma Basic. After about 4 months, there was a lasting improvement. Today the leg feels warm, the pulse in the foot is distinctly tangible. Ms. S. can once again go on longer walks. The costs for the remedy have been covered by the insurance board since Padma Basic is on the list of specialties in Switzerland.

(Source: Information text from SAT 1, TV Station)

DIABETES MELLITUS– IMPROVED THROUGH PADMA BASIC

At the Tibetan Medicine Congress in Washington of 1998, Dr. Dorjee Rabten Neshar from the Tibetan Medicine Center of Bangalore (India) explained how Tibetan physicians provide successful therapy for diabetes with herbs. However, as the practice shows, through its antioxidant potential Padma Basic can also contribute to controlling diabetes mellitus—above all, the type II (late-onset diabetes), which frequently occurs together with circulatory disorders. (Any attempt of this type should definitely be discussed first with the treating physician.)

PADMA BASIC PROMOTES THE HEALING OF WOUNDS

In response to my appeal to the readers, two interesting letters were sent to me on the topic of diabetes. In the first case, Mr. K. of G. reported that his wife, who suffered from diabetes, had a resulting leg wound healed in 1998.

A blister had formed on her big toe as a result of walking; because of her high blood-sugar values, this turned into an open wound that did not heal for months. The circulation in the entire leg became increasingly poor, which is why even an amputation was being considered.

After Mr. K. had learned about Padma Basic from the Fliege show, his wife immediately began taking it. After the first 400 tablets, Ms. K. felt that she no longer had cold feet. The capillary circulation had begun to function once again, and the wound on the foot slowly began to close. After taking about 800 tablets of Padma Basic and a treatment period of approximately 7 months, the toe had healed completely. Ms. K.'s family doctor could hardly believe her eyes—she had reckoned with an amputation.

(The author has a copy of the medical findings of this case.)

PADMA BASIC HAS MADE MY LIFE MORE DELIGHTFUL

In the second case, Mr. H. of M. wrote that he began taking Padma Basic as an insulin-dependent diabetic in October of 2001. As early as the beginning of December, his glucose levels began to slowly decrease, with the result that Mr. H. now can inject 5-7 fewer units of insulin per day.

"Padma Basic" he says, "has made my life more delightful since little dietary sins like a piece of cake or chocolate almost do not influence my levels at all."

(Translation of original letter to the author)

Heart disease is the leading cause of death among diabetics, with a two-to-four fold risk over non-diabetics. The annual rate of lower-limb amputations performed on diabetics in the US is 82,000 (an average from years 1997-1999).

As a result of overeating and lack of exercise, type II diabetes is occurring with increasing frequency. A serious change in our way of thinking has become necessary in relation to our Western lifestyle.

At the same time, the statement of ancient original Tibetan texts come to mind: They say that Tibetan medicine offers remedies for "new plagues of modern times." In one form or another, this may actually prove to be true.

TIBETAN MEDICATIONS IN THE WEST

QUALITY CONTROL AND PERSPECTIVES FOR THE FUTURE

If we are to succeed in building a bridge between Eastern methods of healing and Western medicine, ways of testing the quality and effectiveness of Tibetan remedies in standardized procedures must be found. In the long run, there is no way around this. H.H. the Dalai Lama, as he has repeatedly emphasized in his many visits to the West, also has this perspective.

IN HARMONY WITH THE MODERN WORLD

The medical formulas of *Padma* are continually subjected to clinical and experimental studies in the practice. Such test series form the scientific basis for a broad-based application of Tibetan medications within the scope of established Western medicine. The Viennese biophysicist, who is now the main partner of *Padma*, Dr. Herbert Schwabl, formulated the company's objective in an interview for the *Freies Berlin* radio station in the following way: "We don't want to offer something foreign because it is something foreign; instead, we want to offer it in a way that can be used in a very practical manner by patients, as well as by physicians."[38]

It is important to avoid prejudices and clichés. This is one of the points that the Padma company emphasizes. Tibetan medicine should not be treated like an abstract mystery but as something that functions even "under the cold scientific eye." It is not the placebo effect or some type of foreign spirituality that produces the healing success of Tibetan medicine. Instead, as the practice has shown, this success also stands up to sober studies conducted by conventional medicine. The idea of a holistic approach in no way detracts from this because holistic thinking exists everywhere—both in the West and in the East. So this is not a matter of bringing some type of "new" medicine, namely the Tibetan, to the West; instead, it involves presenting evidence of the real applicability of this old system in a different cultural group. Or, as H.H. the Dalai Lama has said: "You don't have to be a Buddhist to be helped by Tibetan medicine. When it works, then it works everywhere and even under contrary circumstances."[39]

The problem of the quality control of medical remedies in the Western countries must be treated as the primary concern. A patient who seeks help and healing has the right to know precisely what he or she is taking or whether a medicine has been manufactured under controlled conditions. *Padma* also does adequate justice to this issue.

SWISS QUALITY CONTROLS

The raw materials used for the *Padma* remedies correspond with the internationally approved pharmaceutical standards. In terms of purity, the components and amounts of harmful substances must meet certain minimum requirements (according to Swiss pharmacopoeia or food quality). There are constant controls to monitor the pesticide content of plants and plant parts, possible bacterial or mold infection, as well as the amount of heavy metals. If there is the slightest sign of such impurities, the material is destroyed. The use of dyes and preservatives or artificial stabilizers is taboo in the production of *Padma* herbal tablets. They only contain minor amounts of the natural tableting substances of sorbitol and silica. These also exist in the plant kingdom.

In addition to all of this, there is something else that is indispensable in making Tibetan medications—a sensory examination: the smell, taste, and overall impression of the final product should simultaneously meet the requirements of traditional Tibetan medicine. And they actually do meet these requirements, as has been confirmed by the positive evaluations of Tibetan physicians who have inspected the production methods of the *Padma* on site. There are currently even considerations of applying the internationally recognized "Guidelines for Good Manufacturing Practice" (Good Manufacturing Practice = GMP) increasingly in India to facilitate the acceptance of Tibetan remedies throughout the world. As a result, it will be possible in the future to make Tibetan preparations available to a larger group of people in a safe, quality-controlled manner. In this respect, the international research makes an important contribution toward the survival and the continued existence of the ancient Tibetan medicine culture.[40]

NO PROBLEM WITH MERCURY

Unfortunately, a case of mercury contamination in untested "Tibetan jewel pills" was reported by the Swiss media in 2001. Poorly researched press reports gave worried consumers reason to believe that this danger could also apply to Padma Basic. Apart from the fact that *Padma* remedies and teas contain no metallic components whatsoever, *Padma* has always seen it as its responsibility to adapt the Tibetan formulas to the Western standards of safety and quality. Because, according to Dr. Herbert Schwabl: "It is not enough to simply consider the traditional Tibetan medicine as a self-service store for Western needs; we must also accomplish scientific translation work ..." Each batch of *Padma* products is tested to ensure that there is no contamination by heavy metals.

A BRIEF HISTORY OF PADMA, INC.

1965 Peter Badmajew, a descendent of a famous Mongolian-Buryat physician family, brought a collection of Tibetan formulas from the estate of his late father through the Iron Curtain to the West. In Switzerland, he gave these documents to the pharmaceutical entrepreneur Karl Lutz, who had already been interested in this topic for some time. Together, they worked out the first (and only, up to now) indication list for Tibetan medicinal remedies in the West, which was edited by the Study Group of Tibetan Medicine, Zurich. Some of the formulas were made on a trial basis and used by Swiss physicians. Karl Lutz gave his herbal mixtures the name of *Padma*, which reflects the Tibetan word for lotus. The 28th formula of the series attracted attention because of its sensational success.

1969 Encouraged by the positive echo from medical groups, Karl Lutz established the company *Padma* in Zurich, where the production of two Tibetan medicines according to strict quality guidelines is initiated.

1970 The formula No. 179 (Padma Lax) is approved for sale by the IKS (= Intercantonal Control Office for Medicines, the Swiss FDA).

1978 Approval of formula No. 28 (Padma Basic) by the Swiss FDA. The numbering of the medicines follows the old list of formulas.

1994 Karl Lutz, now in poor health, turned over the management of the *Padma* to his close collaborator, the Viennese biophysicist Dr. Herbert Schwabl. Dr. Schwabl had headed the first far-ranging studies on the mechanism of action in Tibetan medicinal remedies.

1998 After the death of Karl Lutz in 1995, Dr. Schwabl obtained the majority of *Padma.* That same year, Padma Basic was approved in Switzerland as a health-insurance medication. This approval was preceded by vehement bureaucratic resistance.

1999 The company moved to the new office building in Schwerzenbach. Modernization of the production plant in Wetzikon.
Four new tea mixtures (*Padma Teas*), also composed according to the traditional Tibetan guidelines, complement the medicinal remedy program.

2001 *Padma* expanded distribution of *Padma* products to North America by collaborating with EcoNugenics, a US-based company that shares the same vision of integrating traditional medical wisdom with solid scientific research.

2001-2003 *Padma* introduced to the market a total of 14 additional remedies, based on ancient original Tibetan formulas—initially in the Swiss Canton of Appenzell Ausserrhoden.

Today Padma Basic can be obtained in Canada and the USA, as well as in nine European countries. Whether it is an over-the-counter medicinal remedy or whether it is a food supplement—as it is in countries like the USA, Canada, Austria, and the Netherlands—depends upon the approval conditions of the respective country.

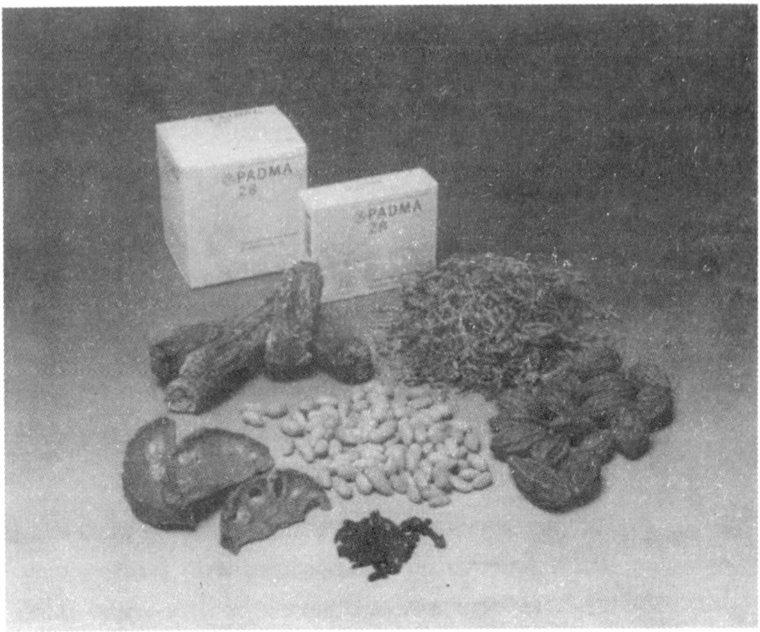

Padma Basic raw herbs

EPILOG: THE SITUATION OF MEDICINE TODAY

The cynical sentence: "Anyone who feels well is not necessarily healthy, just not properly examined," may appear a bit exaggerated in view of the very useful field of preventive medicine. However, one look at our Western health system is enough to provide evidence for the truth at its heart.

While increasingly more people are sent to conventional medical "analysis" and treatment today, we are still very far removed from healing or even achieving a deeper understanding of many of the "scourges of humanity," including cancer and AIDS. Whether the enormous efforts in terms of time and means stands in an appropriate relationship to the success that has been achieved is yet to be seen. The same applies to whether the rapid advances in gene technology will only prove to be a blessing.

THE FORGOTTEN HERITAGE

Western medicine's abandonment of a holistic way of looking at the human beings has led to a mechanistic perspective of sickness and health; and it has since nurtured the idea that every disorder of the "human machine" can be eliminated through the appropriate interventions by modern high-tech medicine.

That this is not the case is proved by a constantly growing host of unnerved patients who feel that they have been left alone with their problems and needs and therefore are increasingly attracted to the so-called alternative methods of healing.

Why has this happened?

As children of the 21st Century, the scientific-technological age, we tend to consider anything that does not fit into the familiar structure of rational explanations to be backwards, primitive, and therefore superfluous. This applies to unfamiliar customs and traditions, as well as the field of medicine. At the same time, we tend to overlook the blinders that this linear way of thinking has put on us.

In our day and age, only "logical" explanations are accepted for medical findings. All of the facts should be comprehendible according to the rules of experimental presentation of the evidence. Since Aristotle, Western culture has been moving on this well-worn track, and only now are we slowly beginning to recognize its treacherousness.

The model of logic, systematics, and objective provability is being increasingly subjected to critical questioning. Knowledge that is called "mystical" is quite unexpectedly receiving a "real" background through new research methods. At the same time, these fields range from microbiology to the revolutionary chaos research.

DIALOG INSTEAD OF MONOLOG

The disregard of folk medicine's knowledge on the part of the university medicine had long prevented any insight into the functioning and backgrounds of traditional system of healing. In the course of the growing interest in foreign cultural groups, a striving for integration and a mutual exchange has also become apparent in medicine.

Especially the study of Asian methods of healing, such as Tibetan medicine, are offering us the opportunity to profit from this enormous source of knowledge, to make it understandable for us in the West, and also to make some of it useable in the West. An evaluation according to scientific criteria is not in contradiction to this approach as long as it is done without prejudice and occurs in consideration of the characteristics of the respective cultural group.

In the process, we should not overlook the fact that much of what appears inexplicable to us today may already be celebrated tomorrow as a sensational new discovery. For example, the Indian tribes of North America had no problem healing scurvy because the cause of this vitamin-deficiency illness that was so feared by the Western explorers was very clear to them. The "white man" ignored this knowledge. When vitamin C was ultimately "discovered" and chemically imitated, the American Indian healers explained that natural vitamin C possessed a different quality and healing effect than synthetic ascorbic acid, even if this could not be seen under the microscope. Their universal understanding of things permitted no other conclusion. Scientists also considered this claim to be nonsense for a long time until special experiments in the 1970s determined a fundamental biochemical difference between natural and artificial vitamin C and were able to scientifically "prove it" for the first time.[41]

CHANGING OUR WAY OF THINKING AND A NEW ORIENTATION

To put it in clear terms: The accomplishments of modern emergency medicine, surgery, and the control of epidemics are remarkable and, used properly, undoubtedly beneficial. Our Western medical professionals do excellent work. However, this can hardly obscure the fact that the procedures of conventional medicine are less effective for a large number of disorders, especially chronic ailments.

It has been proved that almost 50% of all prescribed chemical medications are never taken by the patients because of actual or feared side-effects. At the same time, the cases of iatrogenic (which means actually caused by the conventional medical treatment) diseases are on the rise.

Consequently, the approach of the future cannot consist of cultivating the differences between conventional medicine and the traditional naturopathy; instead, we must discover which type of treatment promises the greatest degree of success with the least amount of risk in the individual cases.

In order to accomplish this, all of the participants must be willing to enter into a discussion and work together. The striving for profits and academic distinctions must become secondary. The principle of "whoever heals is right" must be given its due respect. A medicine that presents itself as a closed system without the willingness to explore new dimensions will serve neither the sick human being nor itself.

In addition to the Western "evidence-based medicine," which is supported by proof and experimental facts, there is also an empiric medicine whose knowledge is based upon the tangible success of its use over a period of centuries and longer throughout the world. Creating a fruitful and respectful cooperation between the representatives of both orientations should be the objective of future research and practice.

The International Congress for Tibetan Medicine, which was held in 1998 in Washington and provided the opportunity for experts and interested individuals from all parts of the world to exchange their knowledge and their practical experiences, can be considered exemplary for these efforts.

Tashi Deleg—May you be well!
(Traditional Tibetan greeting)

APPENDIX

ACKNOWLEDGEMENTS

For their advisory help and support, I would particularly like to thank:

The staff of the pharmacy *Stadelhofen-Apotheke*, Zurich, Switzerland

Mr. Reinhold Gabriel of the company *Sanova Ges.mbH*, Vienna, Austria

And, finally, my family and especially my husband. Without his assistance, I would have been defenseless against all of the computer's wiles.

NOTES AND REFERENCES

Introduction: The Wisdom of the Medicine-Buddha

1 Cf. in: *Medizin Zeitung—Schweizer Fachzeitung fuer das Gesundheitswesen*, 6th ed., 3/ March 1999: V. Hylton, *"Tibetische Medizin"*

2 Cf. in: *Medical Tribune*, 30th ed., 50/Dec. 11, 1998: *"Erster Weltkongress fuer tibetische Medizin—Die Globalisierung der Naturmedizin"*

Tibetan Remedies—The Knowledge of Healing

3 *Das Wissen vom Heilen*, Haupt-Verlag, Zurich, 1998, pg. 175-183

4 Ibid, p. 35ff.

5 Quoted according to *Pharma-Time* No. 12/1998: *"Tibetische Medizin—Weltkongress mit Oesterreichischer Beteiligung"*

6 Cf. *Medizin Zeitung—Schweizer Fachzeitung fuer das Gesundheitswesen*, 6th ed., 4/April 1999, V. Hylton: *Tibetische Medizin*, Part 2

7 Cf. Franz Reichle: *Das Wissen vom Heilen*, p. 138ff.

8 Ibid, p. 19

Padma Basic—Messenger of a Gentle Medicine

9 Cf. Franz Reichle: *Das Wissen vom Heilen*, p. 106ff.

10 Cf. *Scientific studies and analyses on the effect of Tibetan multi-substance mixtures* (see listing below)

Padma Basic—Motor of the Immune System

11 Cf. Harman, D.: "Free Radical Theory of Aging: History" in: *Free Radicals and Aging*, eds. I. Ement and B. Chance, Basel, Switzerland, 1992

12 Cf. Fritz Albert Popp: *Die Botschaft der Nahrung*, Verlag Zweitausendeins 1999

13 Cf. in: *Scientific studies and analyses on the effect of Tibetan multi-substance mixtures* (see listing below)

14 Cf. Stephan Kolb, Fichtestrasse 39, 91054 Erlangen, Germany: Radio Interview for the station *Sender Freies Berlin: "... wem das Kraut gewachsen ist. Asiatische Heilkraeuter auf dem Pruefstand*, SFB, 25-3-2000; p. 9/10

15 Cf. Packer, L.: "Health Effects of Nutritional Antioxidants" in *Free Radical Biol Medic* 1993; 15: 685-686

16 Cf. E. Asshauer: *Gesund bleiben mit der Heilkunst der Tibeter*, Stuttgart 1999, p. 134

17 Cf. in: *Scientific studies and analyses on the effect of Tibetan multi-substance mixtures* (see listing below)

Padma Basic and Arteriosclerosis

18 Cf. Franz Reichle: *Das Wissen vom Heilen*, p. 106ff.

19 Ibid, p. 108/109

20 Cf. in: *Scientific studies and analyses on the effect of Tibetan multi-substance mixtures* (see listing below)

21 Ibid

22 Ibid

Padma Basic and Cancer

23 Cf. Siegfried Block: *Die grosse Chance*, Munich 1982, p. 195ff.

24 Ibid, s. 76ff.

25 Cf. Franz Reichle: *Das Wissen vom Heilen*, p. 120-122

Tibetan Medicines—Also Good for the Soul?

26 Cf. Geoff Deehan: "The Healing Power of the Psyche"—ORF documentary from 4/8/1993 (VATV London), German translation in: *ORF-Nachlese* 1993; 7: 16-20

27 Ibid, s. 17

28 Ibid, s. 18

29 Ibid, s. 18

Additional Areas of Use for Padma Basic

30 Cf. Franz Reichle: *Das Wissen vom Heilen*, p. 136-201

31 Cf. in: *Scientific studies and analyses on the effect of Tibetan multi-substance mixtures* (see listing below)

32 Cf. E. Asshauer: *Gesund bleiben mit der Heilkunst der Tibeter*, Stuttgart 1999, s. 134

33 Ibid, p. 139

34 Cf. in: *Scientific studies and analyses on the effect of Tibetan multi-substance mixtures* (see listing below)

35 Cf. in: *APAMED (*the online information system for health professionals*)* of 11/9/1998: *Tibetische Medizin 2—Jede "Schule" hat ihre Vorteile*

36 Cf. in: *Scientific studies and analyses on the effect of Tibetan multi-substance mixtures* (see listing below)

Padma Lax

37 Cf. *B & K Kommunikation*, Thurngasse 8/10, 1090 Vienna, Austria, of 11/11/1998: *"Erster Internationaler Kongress ueber Tibetische Medizin in Washington D.C.—Westliche Forscher bestaetigen die Wirksamkeit Tibetischer Kraeutermischungen,"* as well as no. 36 (see above)

Tibetan Medicine in the West

38 Quoted according to Stephan Kolb, Fichtestrasse 39, 91054 Erlangen, Germany: Radio Interview for the station *Freies Berlin*: *"... wem das Kraut gewachsen ist. Asiatische Heilkraeuter auf dem Pruefstand,"* SFB, 25-3-2000; p. 1/2

39 Cf. Ibid, p. 2/3

40 Cf.: *"Zur Qualitaet der Tibetischen Rezepturen,"* © 2000 by *Padma, Inc.*, Schwerzenbach, Switzerland

41 Cf. H. J. Stammel: *Das Heilwissen der Indianer*, Reinbeck 1986, p. 49

RECOMMENDED READING

Aschoff, Juergen / Rosing, Ina: *Tibetan Medicine—East meets West, West meets East*, Fabri Verlag, Ulm (Germany), 1997

Dalai Lama / Hopkins Jeffrey: *Kindness—Clarity—Insight*, Snow Lion Publications, Inc., Ithaca NY (USA) 1984

Dalai Lama / Hopkins Jeffrey: *The Dalai Lama at Harvard: Lectures on the Buddhist Path to Peace*, Snow Lion Publications, Inc., Ithaca NY (USA) 1989

Donden, Yeshi: *Healing from the Source*, Snow Lion Publications, Inc., Ithaca NY (USA) 2000

Dunkenberger, Thomas: *Tibetan Healing Handbook*, Lotus Press, Twin Lakes (USA) 2000

Fundamentals of Tibetan Medicine, Tibetan Medical & Astro Institute: Dharamsala (India), 2002

Horrigan, Bonnie: *Robert Thurman, Gifts from Tibetan Medicine*, Alternative Therapies 2002; 9/1: 85-93

Kelly, Petra K./Bastian, Gert (ed.): *The Anguish of Tibet*, Parallax PR 1991

Losang, Ragpay: *The Tibetan Book of Healing*, Lotus Press, Twin Lakes (USA) 2000

Samel, Gerti: *Tibetan Medicine*, Little, Brown & Company, London 2001

Sither, Bradley Tamdin: *Principles of Tibetan Medicine*, HarperCollins Publishers, Glasgow (UK) 2000

DVD and Film:

DVD (European Standard PAL): Reichle, Franz (ed.): *The Knowledge of Healing*, 2003

Film (European Standard VHS-PAL): Reichle Franz (ed.): *The Knowledge of Healing*, Fox Video (UK)

IN GERMAN:

Amipa-Desam, Tendhon: *Klassische Tibetische Medizin*, Ehrenwirth Verlag, Munich (Germany) 2000

Asshauer, Egbert: *Heilkunst vom Dach der Welt–Tibets sanfte Medizin*, Herder Verlag, Freiburg (Germany) 1993

Asshäuer, Egbert: *Gesund bleiben mit der Heilkunst der Tibeter*, Thieme Verlag, Stuttgart (Germany) 1999

Choedrak Tenzin: *Ganzheitlich leben–Der Leibarzt des Dalai Lama ueber Vorbeugung und Therapie von Krankheiten*, Herder/Spektrum, Freiburg (Germany) 1994

Clifford, Terry: *Tibetische Heilkunst*, O.W. Barth Verlag, Munich (Germany) 1986

Craig, M.: *Traenen ueber Tibet. Der erschuetternde Bericht ueber die Unterdrueckung der Tibeter and die Zerstoerung ihrer alten Kultur*, Scherz Verlag, Bern (Switzerland)/Munich (Germany) 1993

Fliege, Juergen / Ohler Walter (ed.): *Sanfte Medizin bei Fliege–alles ist moeglich*, BIO Ritter Verlag, Tutzing (Germany) 2002

Kraemer, Claus: *Traditionelle Tibetische Medizin*, Midena Verlag, Munich (Germany) 2000

Reichle, Franz (ed.): *Das Wissen vom Heilen*, Oesch-Verlag, Zurich, revised edition 2003 (US version is planned), book to the film: Reichle Franz (ed.): *The Knowledge of Healing*, (European Standard VHS-PAL) Fox Video (UK)

Tsewang J. Tsarong / Meyer, F. / Asshauer, E.: *Tibet und seine Medizin–2500 Jahre Heilkunst*, Pinguin Verlag, Innsbruck (Austria) 1992

SCIENTIFIC STUDIES AND ANALYSES ON THE EFFECT OF TIBETAN MULTI-SUBSTANCE MIXTURES

(Selection)

Altermatt R., von Felten A.: *"In-vitro-Untersuchungen mit Padma 28: Hemmung der Thrombozytenfunktion"*
Schweiz Z Ganzheitsmed 1992; 4 (Suppl 1): 7-12

Asshauer E.: *"Padma 28—eine tibetische Kraeutermischung als Immunmodulator"*
Naturheilpraxis 1991; 44: 138-141

Asshauer E.: *"Tibetische Kraeuterpillen und Padma 28 bei westlichen Patienten"*
Paracelsus report 1998; 5/98: 55-58

Asshauer E.: *"Padma 28—ein tibetisches Heilmittel—Arzneimittelstudie"*
Naturheilpraxis 1987; 40: 1134-1143

Bainerman-Fishman R.: *"Antioxidants and phytotherapy"*
The Lancet 1994; 344: 1356

Becker S.: *"Chronische Krankheitsprozesse: Pathogenese und Behandlung. Die Perspektive der Phytopharmakologie von Vielstoff-Kraeuterpraeparaten"*
Schweiz Z Ganzheitsmed 1997; 7(8: 350-352

Becker S.: *"Revealing the art of the medicine Buddha"—First International Congress for Tibetan Medicine, Washington D.C., November 7-9, 1998.*
Schweiz Z Ganzheitsmed 1999; 11/3

Bernacka K., Sierakowski St., Brzosko W.J.: *"PADMA 28 in the therapy of rheumatoid arthritis; A 6-months clinical and laboratory study"*
Abstract; 4th Interscience World Conference on Inflammation, Geneva, April 1991

Bommeli C., Bohnsack R., and Kolb C.: *"Praxiserfahrungen mit einem Vielstoffpraeparat aus der tibetischen Heilkunde"*
Erfahrungsheilkunde 2001; 50/11: 745-756

Briviba K., Sies H., in *Frei B.* (ed.): *"Natural antioxidants in human health and disease"*
Academic Press, San Diego 1994: 107-128

Brzosko W.J., Jankowski A.: *"Padma 28 bei chronischer Hepatitis B: Klinische und immunologische Wirkungen"*
Schweiz Z Ganzheitsmed 1992; 7/8 (Suppl 1): 13-14

Brzosko W.J., Jankowski A.: *"Influence of PADMA 28 and gamma-linolenic acid on clinical and immunological parameters in patients with CAH type B"*
Abstract; FalkSymposium, Basel, Switzerland, September 10-13, 1992

Brzosko W. J. et al: *"Influence of Padma 28 and thymus extract on clinical and laboratory parameters of children with juvenile chronic arthritis"*
Int J Immunotherapy 1991; 7: 143-147

Brzosko W.J., Debski R., Wisniewska W., Jankowski A.: *"Treatment with PADMA 28 of childr en with chronic active hepatitis infected with HBV"*
Abstract; 19th Int'l Congress of Pediatrics, Paris, July 23-28, 1989

Brzosko W.J., Gladysz A., Juszczyk J.: *"PADMA 28 in der Behandlung der chronisch aktiven Hepatitis. PADMA 28 in the tr eatment of chronic active hepatitis"*
Biologische Medizin 1986; 15: 300-305

Cottier H., Holdler J., and Kraft R.: *"Oxidative stress: Pathogenetic mechanisms"*
Forsch Komplementaermed 1995; 2: 223-239

Draebaek H., Mehlsen J.. Himmelstrup H., and Winther K.: *"A botanical compound, Padma 28, increases walking distance in stable intermittent claudication*
Angiology 1993; 44: 863-867
Forsch Komplementaermed 1995; 2/5: 240-245

Fishman R.H.B.: *"Antioxidants and phytotherapy"*
The Lancet 1994; 344:1356

Flueck H, Bubb Ph.: *"Eine lamaistische Rezeptformel zur Behandlung der chronischen Verstopfung"*
Schweiz Rundschau Med (PRAXIS) 1970; 59: 1190-1193

Ginsburg I., Sadovnik M., Sallon S., Milo-Goldtwog I., Mechoulam R., Breuer A., Gibbs D., Varani J., Roberts S., Cleator E., and Singh N.: *"Padma 28, a traditional Tibetan herbal preparation inhibits the respiratory burst in human neutrophils, the killing of epithelial cells by mixtures of oxidants and pro-inflammatory agonists and peroxidation of lipids"*
Inflammopharmacology 1999; 7/1: 47-62

Gladysz A., Juszczyk J., and Brzosko W.: *"Influence of Padma 28 on patients with chronic active hepatitis type B"*
Phytother Res 1993; 7: 244-247

Haessig A., Liang Wen-Xi, Schwabl H., and Stampfli K.: *"Flavoine und Tannine: Pflanzliche Antioxidanzien mit Vitamincharakter"*
Schweiz Z Ganzheitsmed 1997; 9 (Suppl 4): 171-175

Haessig A., Liang Wen-Xi, and Stampfli K.: *"Neuroendokrine Steuerung der Immunreaktionen"*
Schweiz Z Ganzheitsmed 1996; 8 (Suppl 5): 231-233

Haessig A., Hodler J., Liang W.X., and Stampfli K.: *"Neuere nutritive and phytotherapeutische Behandlungsmoeglichkeiten"*
Schweiz Z Ganzheitsmed 1992; 4 (Suppl 1): 15-19

Hasik J. et al.: *"Efficacy of Padma 28 and Padma 137 in treatment of patients with peptic duodenal ulcer" (in Polish)*
Nowiny Lekarskie (Poznan/Poland) 1992; 2: 40-44

Hertog M.G.L.: *"Antioxidative Flavonoide in der Nahrung: Herzinfarkt- und Karzinomrisiken"*
Forsch Komplementaermed 1995; 2: 283-288

Hryniewiecki L., Brzosko W.J., Klincewicz H., Stachowiak Cz.: *"Treatment of patients with active liver cirrhosis with PADMA 28".*
Lecture at the Int'l Symposium "Chronic Disease Processes: Pathogenesis and Treatment. The perspective of herbal multicompound preparations," University Roskilde/ Denmark, September 28-29, 1997

Huerlimann F.: *"Behandlung peripherer Durchblutungsstoerungen mit Padma 28—Erfahrungen ueber 15 Jahre"*
Schweiz Z Ganzheitsmed 1992; 4 (Suppl 1): 20-21

Huerlimann F.: *"Eine lamaistische Rezeptformel zur Behandlung der peripheren arteriellen Verschlusskrankheit"*
Schweiz Rsch Med 1979; 67: 1407-1409

Jankowski A., Jankowska R., and Brzosko W.J.: *"Behandlung infektanfaelliger Kinder mit Padma 28"*
Schweiz Z Ganzheitsmed 1992; 4 (Suppl 1): 22-23

Jankowski S., Jankowski A., Zielinski S., and Walzuk M.: *"Influence of Padma 28 on the spontaneous bactericidal activity of blood serum in children suffering from recurrent infections of the respiratory tract"*
Phytother Res 1991; 5: 120-123

Jankowksi A., Prusek W., Brzosko W.J.: *"Treatment of prone to infection children with natural immuno correctors"*
Abstract; 19th Int'l Congress of Pediatrics, Paris, July 23-28, 1989

Jankowski A., Drabbik E., Szyszko Z., Stasiewicsz W., and Brzosko W.J.: *"Die Behandlung rezidivierender Atemwegsinfektionen bei Kindern durch Aktivierung des Immunsystems"*
Therapiewoche Schweiz 1986: 2: 25-32

Kieffer F.: *"Eisenüberladung und oxidativer Stress"*
Forsch Komplementaermed 1995; 2: 259-267

Korwin-Piotrowska T. et al: *"Experience of Padma 28 in Multiple Sclerosis"*
Phytother Res 1992; 6: 133-136

Liang W.X., Stampfli K., and Haessig A.: *"Therapeutische Wirkungsmechanismen komplexer Phytopharmaka am Beispiel von Padma 28"*
Schweiz Z Ganzheitsmed 1992; 4 (Suppl 1): 24-34

Mansfeld H. J.: *"Beeinflussung rezidivierender Atemwegsinfekte bei Kindern durch Immunstimulation"*
Therapeutikon 1988; 2: 707-712

Matzner Y., Sallon S.: *"The effect of Padma 28, a traditional Tibetan herbal preparation, on human neutrophil function"*
J Clin Lab Immunol 1995; 46: 13-23

Mehlsen J., Drabaeck H., Peterson J. R., and Winther K.: *"Der Effekt einer tibetischen Kraeutermischung (Padma 28) auf die Gehstrecke bei stabiler Claudicatio intermittens"*
Forsch Komplementaermedizin 1995; 2: 240-245 and
Angiology 1993; 44: 863-867

Moeslinger T., Friedl R., Volf I., Brunner M., Koller E., and Spieckermann P.G.: *"Inhibition of inducible nitric oxide synthesis by the herbal preparation Padma 28 in macrophage cell line"*
Can J Physiol Pharmacol 2000; 78/11: 861-866

Muehlbauer R.C.: "Fördern ungesättigte Fettsäuren den oxidativen Stress?"
Forsch Komplementaermed 1995; 2: 268-277

Prusek W. et al: "Immunostimulation in recurrent respiratory tract infections therapy in children"
Arch Immunol Ther Exp 1987; 35: 289-302

Ryan M.: *"Efficacy of the Tibetan treatment for arthritis"*
Soc. Sci. Med. 1997; 44/4: 535-539

Saller R., Kristof O.: *"Padma 28, eine traditionelle tibetische Kraeutermischung"*
Internist Praxis 1997; 37: 408-412

Saller R., Kristof O., and Reichling J.: *"Padma 28, ein traditionelles und modernes Phytotherapeutikum"*
Zs Phytother 1997; 6: 323-331

Sallon S., Ben-Arye E., Davidson R., Shapiro H., Ginsberg G., and Ligumsky M.: *"A novel treatment for constipation-predominant irritable bowel syndrome using Padma Lax, a Tibetan herbal formula"*
Digestion 2002; 65: 161-171; S. Karger AG, Basel

Sallon S., Beer G., Rosenfeld J., Anner H., Volcoff D., Ginsberg G., Paltiel O., and Berlatzky Y.: *"The efficacy of Padma 28, a herbal preparation, in the treatment of intermittent claudication: a double-blind study with objective assessment of chronic occlusive arterial disease patients"*
J Vascular Investigation 1998; 4: 129-136

Samochowiec J., Palacz A., Bobnis W., and Lisiecka B.: *"Oscillating potentials of the electroretinogram in the evaluation of the effects of PADMA 28 on lipid metabolism and vascular changes in humans"*
Phytotherapy Research 1992; 6: 200-204

Samochowiec L. et al: *"Wirksamkeitspruefung von Padma 28 bei der Behandlung von Patienten mit chronischen arteriellen Durchblutungsstoerungen (Claudicatio intermittens, Fontaine Stadium II). Part I"*
Herba Pol 1987; 33: 49-61
Polbiophar Reports 1985; 21: 3-40

Samochowiec L. et al.: *"Wirksamkeitsprüfung von Padma 28 bei der Behandlung von Patienten mit Chronischen Arteriellen Durchblutungsstörungen (Claudicatio intermittens, Fontaine Stadium II). Part II"*
Polbiopharm Reports 1987; 22: 3-14

Samochowiec L., Wojcicki J.: *"Effect of PADMA 28 on lipid endoperoxides formation"*
Herba Pol 1987; 33/3: 219-222 and Polbiopharm Reports 1987; 22: 15-19

Schleicher P.: *"Wirkung von Padma 28 auf das Immunsystem bei Patienten mit Acquired Immunodeficiency Syndrome im Stadium Pre-Aids"*
Schweiz Z Ganzheitsmed 1990; 2: 58-62

Schraeder R., Nachbur M., and Mahler F.: *"Wirksamkeit von Padma 28 auf die Claudicatio intermittens bei chronisch peripherer arterieller Verschlusskrankheit: Kontrollierte Doppelblindstudie"*
Schweiz Med Wochenschr 1985; 115: 752-756 and Inaugural Dissertation Univ. Bern, Switzerland 1984

Schwabl H.: *"Tibetan medicinc: A question of how West should meet East"*
Tibetan Review, Vol XXXIII/I, January 1998

Schwabl H.: *"Nichtlineare Physik und Systemtheorie: Grundlagen für das Verstaendnis komplexer Wirkmechanismen"*
Schweiz Z Ganzheitsmed 1992; 7/8 (Suppl 1): 41-44

Schwabl H., Klima H.: *"Untersuchungen zur Wirkung eines komplexen Phytotherapeutikums auf die Lichtemission polymorphkerniger Granulozyten in vitro"*
Study report, Atominstitut of the Universities, Vienna, Austria, June 2, 1992 (PhD Thesis published 1994)

Schwabl H. Klima H.: *"Lichtregulation im immunologischen Geschehen am Beispiel eines tibetischen Pflanzenpraeparats*
In: Stacher A., Ganzheitsmedizin–Zweiter Wiener Dialog, ed Facultas Universitaetsverlag, Vienna 1991: 315-320

Smulski H.S., Wojcicki J.: *"Placebokontrollierte Doppelblindstudie zur Wirkung des tibetischen Kraeuterpraeparats Padma 28 auf die Claudicatio intermittens"*
Forsch Komplementaermedizin 1994; 1: 17-26 and Alternative Therapies 1995; 1/3: 44-49

Somoggy S., Schleicher P.: *"Therapie der peripheren arterielle Verschlusskrankheit (PAVK) mit PADMA 28. Teil I: Klinische und Immunologische Wirkung von PADMA 28 beim Patienten mit PAVK im Stadium II a+b nach Fontaine. Teil II: Der Einfluss von PADMA 28 auf das Immunsystem–Messung der Subpopulation der Lymphozyten und Bewertung der Adhaerenz, Motilitaet und Phagozytoserate"*
Study report, Dept of Vascular Surgery, Klinikum rechts der Isar, Techn Universität, Munich/Germany, June 2€ 1990

Stampfli S., Bommeli C., and Schwabl H.: *"Zum antioxidativen und antiinflammatorischen Wirkprofil von Padma 28. Eine Uebersicht"*
Schweiz Z Ganzheitsmed 2001; 13(4): 242-245

Suter M., Richter Ch.: *"Anti- and pro-oxidative properties of PADMA 28, a Tibetan herbal formulation"*
Redox Report 2000; 5/1: 17-22

Ueberall F., Jenny M., Schwaiger W.: *"The Tibetan remedy PADMA 28 fights tumour cell growth in cell culture"*
European J. Biochem. PS4-050,76, 28th Meeting of the Federation of European Biochemical Societies, October 20-25, 2002, Istanbul, Turkey

Weseler A., Saller R., and Reichling J.: *"Comparative Investigation of the antimicrobial activity of Padma 28 and selected European herbal drugs"*
Forsch Komplementaermed 2002; 9/6: 346-351

Winther K., Kharazmi A., Himmelstrup H., Draback H., and Mehlsen J.: *"Padma 28, a botanical compound, decreased the oxidative burst response of monocytes and improves fibrinolysis in patients with stable intermittent claudication"*
Fibrinolysis 1994; 8 (Suppl 2): 47-49

Wojcicki J., Samochowiec L.: *"Controlled double-blind study of Padma-28 in angina pectoris"*
Herba Pol 1986; 32: 107-114

Zebrowski A, Brzosko WJ, Waszyrowski T, Brykalski M, Iwaszkiewicz J.: *"Immunoscintigraphy in the diagnosis and therapy monitoring in myocarditis"*
Abstract; XII Congress of the European Society of Cardiology, Stockholm, Sweden, Sept. 16-20, 1990

In addition to the above study reports, the author also has professional publications and press texts from *Padma, Inc.*, as well as various reports by satisfied users of Padma Basic.

ADDITIONAL RESOURCES

- North American Distributor of *Padma:*
  www.econugenics.com
  EcoNugenics, Inc.
  2208 Northpoint Parkway
  Santa Rosa, CA 95404
  Phone: (800) 308-5518

- General information about the situation of Tibet,
  www.tibet.com
  the exile Tibetans, Tibetan culture and Tibetan medicine: www.savetibet.org
  www.tibethouse.org

- Information about Tibetan medicine:
  www.amfoundation.org/tibetanmedicine.htm

- Information about integrating ancient medicinal
  www.dreliaz.com
  systems with standard medical treatment:
  Better Health Publishing
  1055 West College Ave. #155
  Santa Rosa, CA 95401
  Phone: (707)521-3362

- Producers of *Padma* products; information about
  www.padma.ch
  the distribution in other countries than the US or Canada:
  Padma, Inc.
  Wiesenstrasse 5
  CH-8603 Schwerzenbach
  Switzerland
  Phone: +41-1-887 00 00
  Fax: +41-1-887-00 99
  Email: mail@padma.ch